MW01132586

The Easiest Way to Learn Human Heart

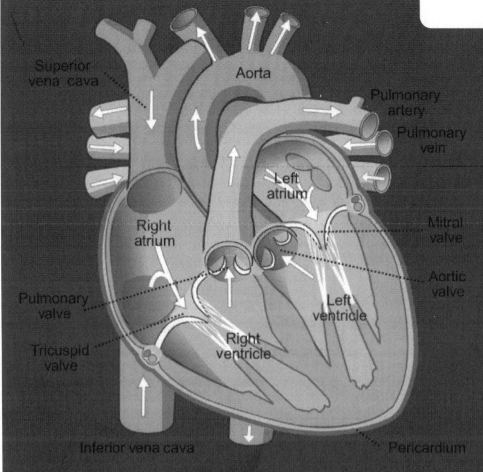

- Superior vena cava
- Aorta
- Pulmonary artery
- Pulmonary vein
- Left atrium
- Mitral valve
- Right atrium
- Aortic valve
- Pulmonary valve
- Left ventricle
- Tricuspid valve
- Right ventricle
- Inferior vena cava
- Pericardium

CARDIOVASCULAR COLORING BOOK FOR ADULT

40 Illustrations	Quiz	Flashcards
Test	Word Search	Crosswords
Matching	Terms Table	Bingo

The Heart

This drawing shows how blood flows through the heart.

Color Me:

The areas of the heart with more oxygen are labeled with an "R". Color these areas RED.

The areas of the heart with less oxygen are labeled with a "B". Color these areas BLUE.

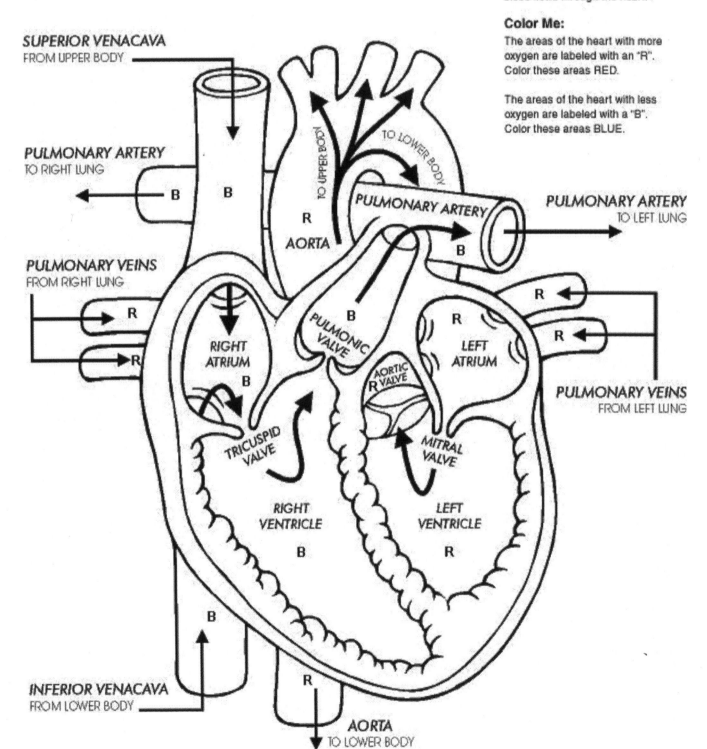

SUPERIOR VENACAVA
FROM UPPER BODY

PULMONARY ARTERY
TO RIGHT LUNG

PULMONARY VEINS
FROM RIGHT LUNG

INFERIOR VENACAVA
FROM LOWER BODY

TO UPPER BODY

TO LOWER BODY

PULMONARY ARTERY

R AORTA

B

PULMONARY ARTERY
TO LEFT LUNG

PULMONARY VEINS
FROM LEFT LUNG

RIGHT ATRIUM

PULMONIC VALVE

LEFT ATRIUM

AORTIC VALVE

TRICUSPID VALVE

MITRAL VALVE

RIGHT VENTRICLE

LEFT VENTRICLE

AORTA
TO LOWER BODY

Name _____ Date _____ Period _____

DIAGRAM OF THE HEART

1. Label the parts of the heart on the diagram (as labeled on the overhead).
2. Use the words from the following word bank.
3. Trace the flow of blood using the red and blue pencils.

Word bank:
Aorta
Superior Vena Cava
Inferior Vena Cava
Right Atrium
Left Atrium

Right Ventricle
Left Ventricle
Tricuspid Valve
Mitral Valve
Apex

Right Pulmonary Artery
Right Pulmonary Vein
Left Pulmonary Artery
Left Pulmonary Veins

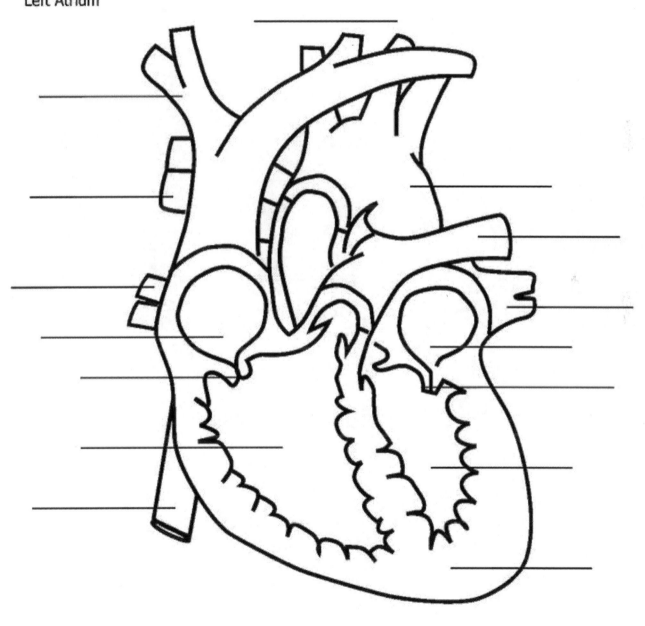

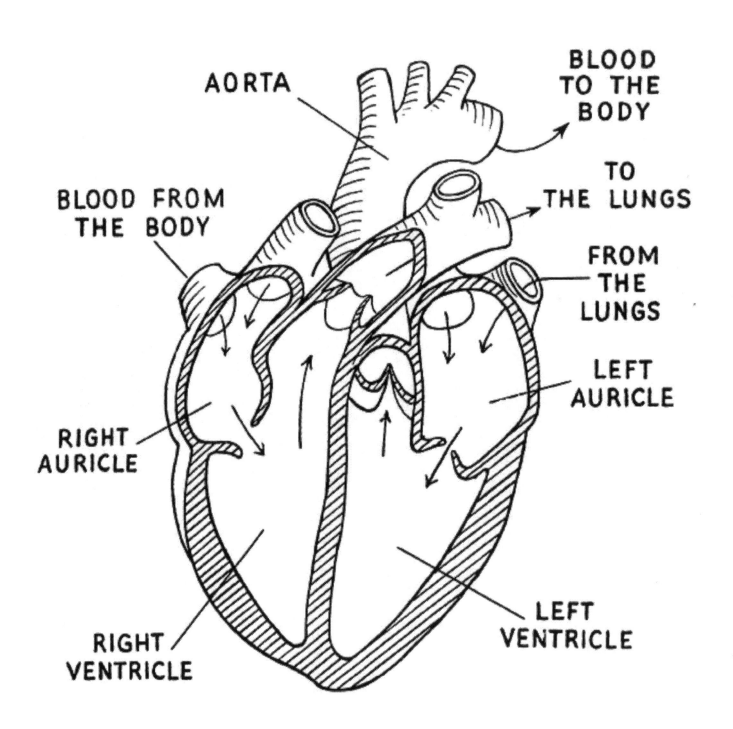

AORTA

BLOOD
TO THE
BODY

BLOOD FROM
THE BODY

TO
THE LUNGS

FROM
THE
LUNGS

LEFT
AURICLE

RIGHT
AURICLE

LEFT
VENTRICLE

RIGHT
VENTRICLE

Color the Anatomy of the Heart

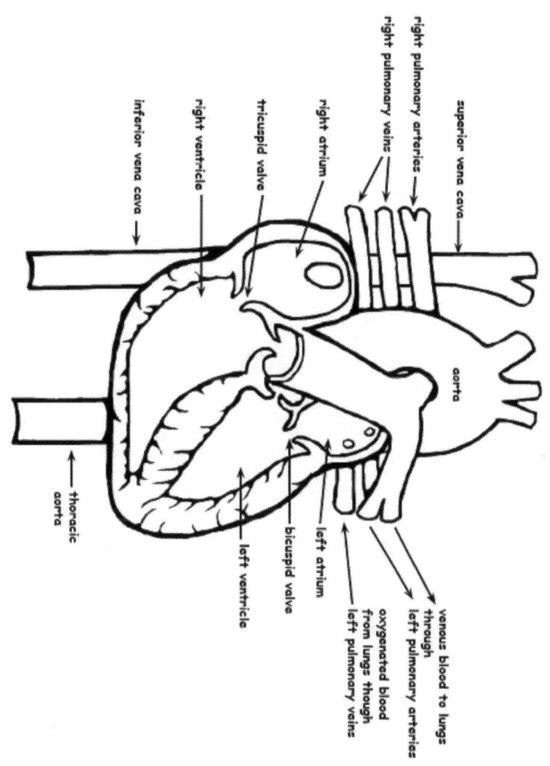

superior vena cava

right pulmonary arteries

right pulmonary veins

right atrium

tricuspid valve

right ventricle

inferior vena cava

thoracic aorta

aorta

left ventricle

bicuspid valve

left atrium

venous blood to lungs through left pulmonary arteries

oxygenated blood from lungs though left pulmonary veins

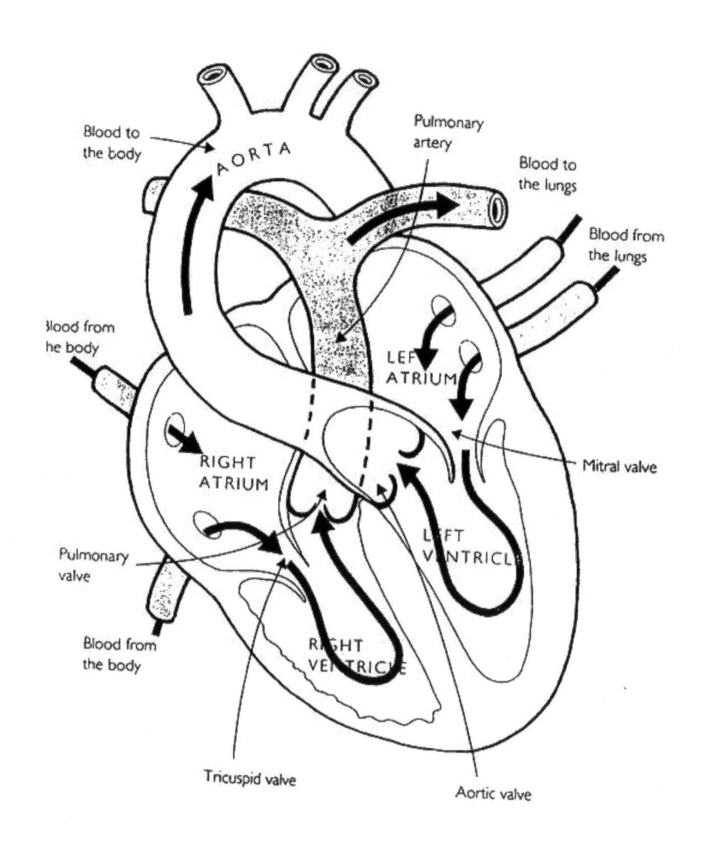

HEART ANATOMY

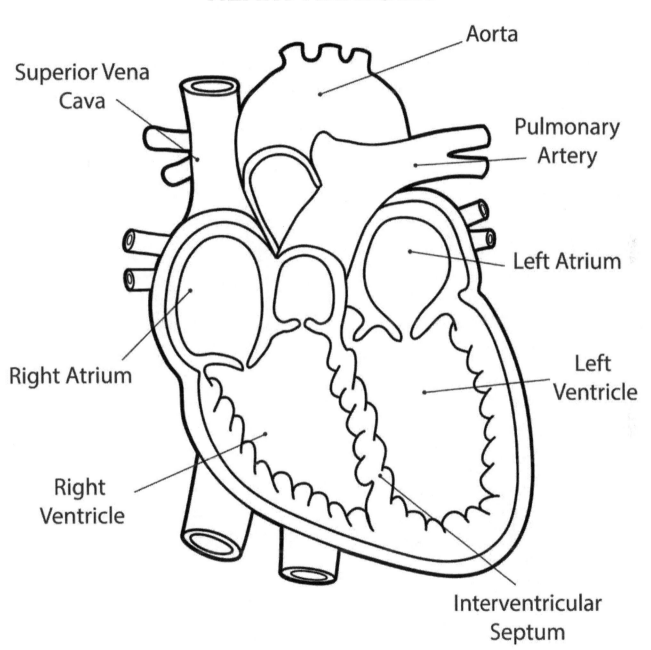

Aorta

Superior Vena
Cava

Pulmonary
Artery

Left Atrium

Right Atrium

Left
Ventricle

Right
Ventricle

Interventricular
Septum

The Human Heart

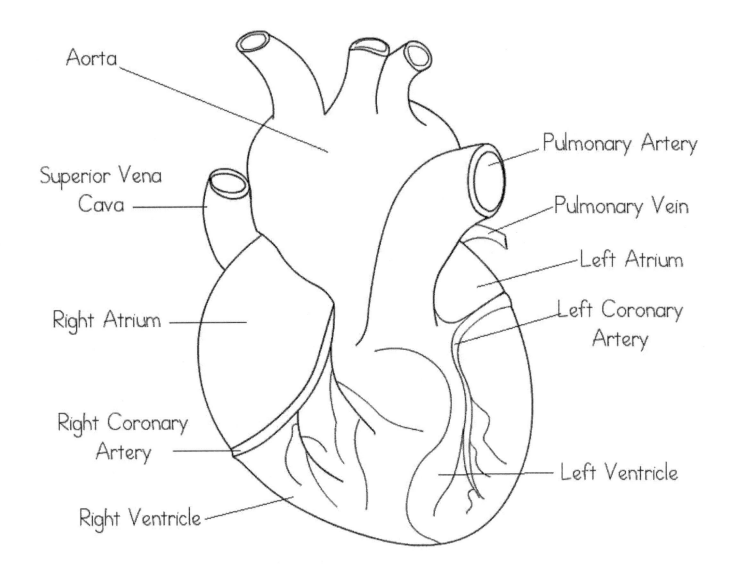

Aorta

Superior Vena Cava

Right Atrium

Right Coronary Artery

Right Ventricle

Pulmonary Artery

Pulmonary Vein

Left Atrium

Left Coronary Artery

Left Ventricle

The Heart

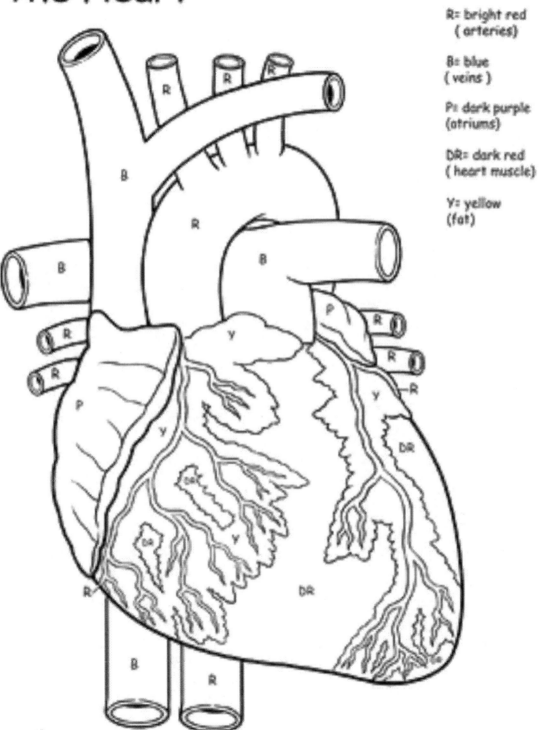

R= bright red
(arteries)

B= blue
(veins)

P= dark purple
(atriums)

DR= dark red
(heart muscle)

Y= yellow
(fat)

Superficial Heart Anatomy (Anterior)

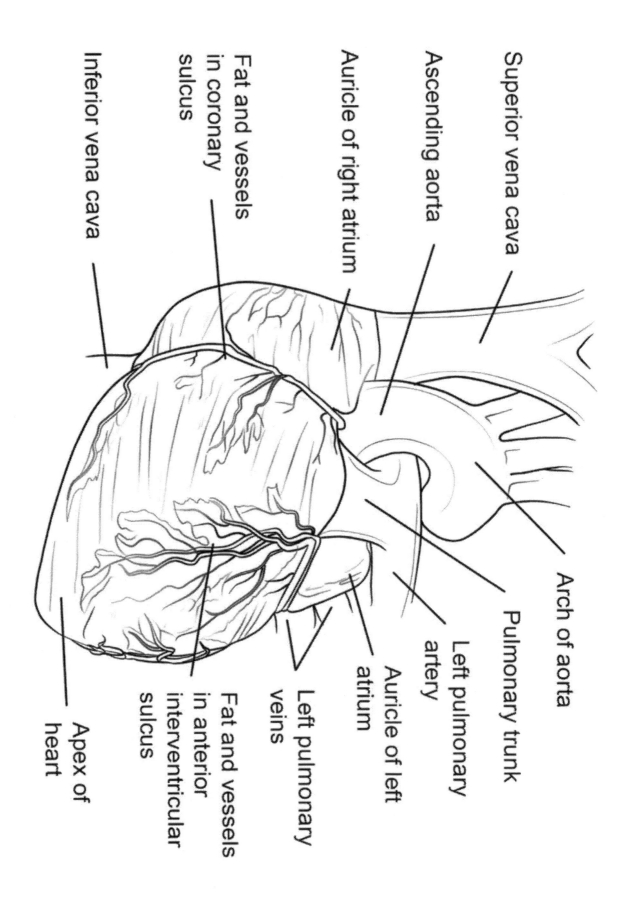

Superior vena cava

Ascending aorta

Auricle of right atrium

Fat and vessels
in coronary
sulcus

Inferior vena cava

Arch of aorta

Pulmonary trunk

Left pulmonary
artery

Auricle of left
atrium

Left pulmonary
veins

Fat and vessels
in anterior
interventricular
sulcus

Apex of
heart

Word Bank
Apex of heart
Arch of aorta
Ascending aorta
Auricle of left atrium
Auricle of right atrium
Fat and vessels in anterior
interventricular sulcus
Fat and vessels in
coronary sulcus
Inferior vena cava
Left pulmonary artery
Left pulmonary veins
Pulmonary trunk
Superior vena cava

Superficial Heart Anatomy (Anterior)

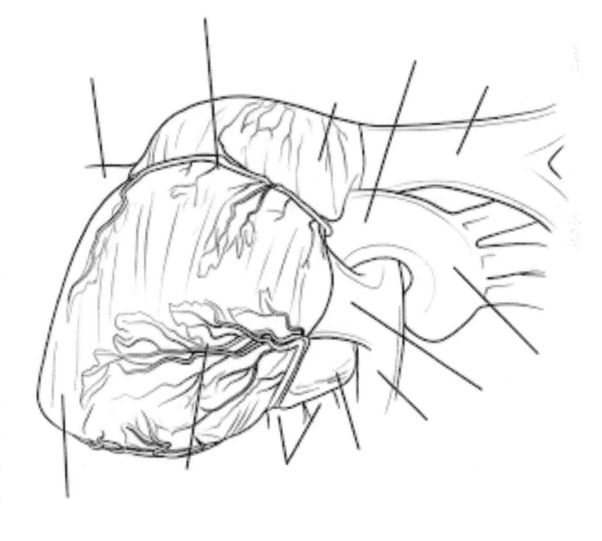

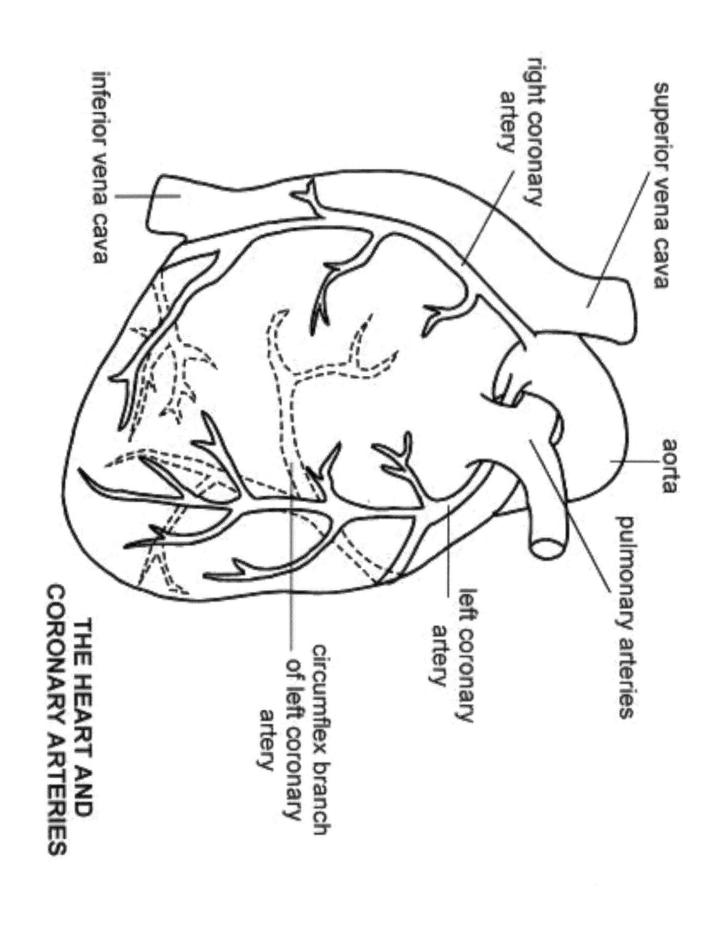

superior vena cava

right coronary
artery

aorta

pulmonary arteries

inferior vena cava

left coronary
artery

circumflex branch
of left coronary
artery

THE HEART AND
CORONARY ARTERIES

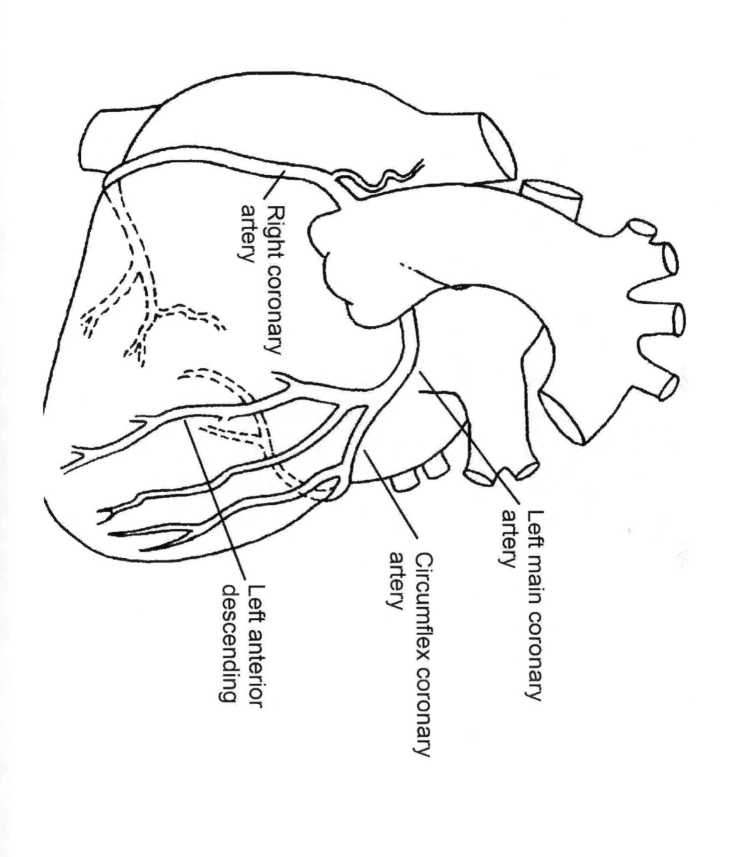

Right coronary artery

Left main coronary artery

Circumflex coronary artery

Left anterior descending

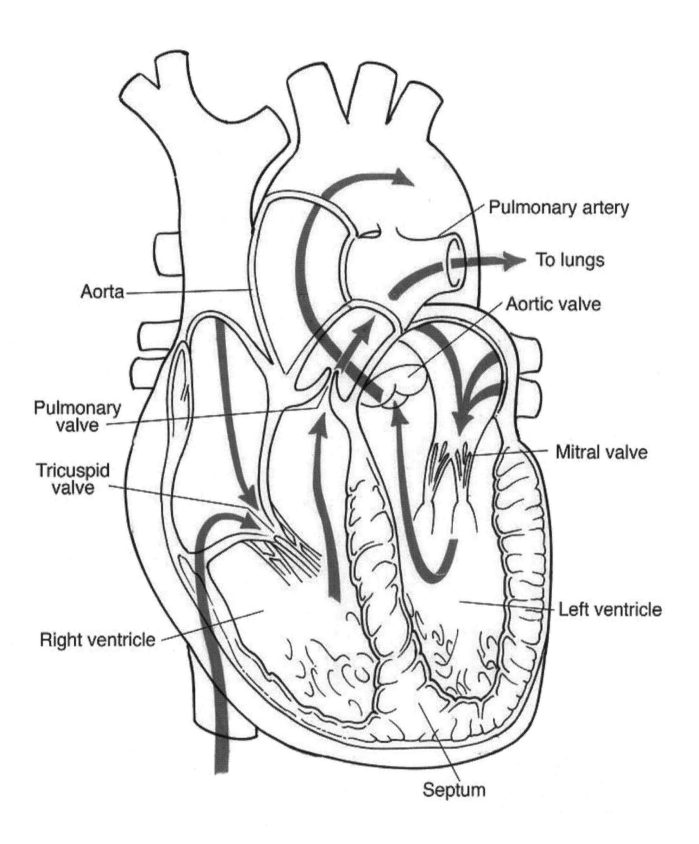

Pulmonary artery

To lungs

Aortic valve

Aorta

Pulmonary valve

Mitral valve

Tricuspid valve

Right ventricle

Left ventricle

Septum

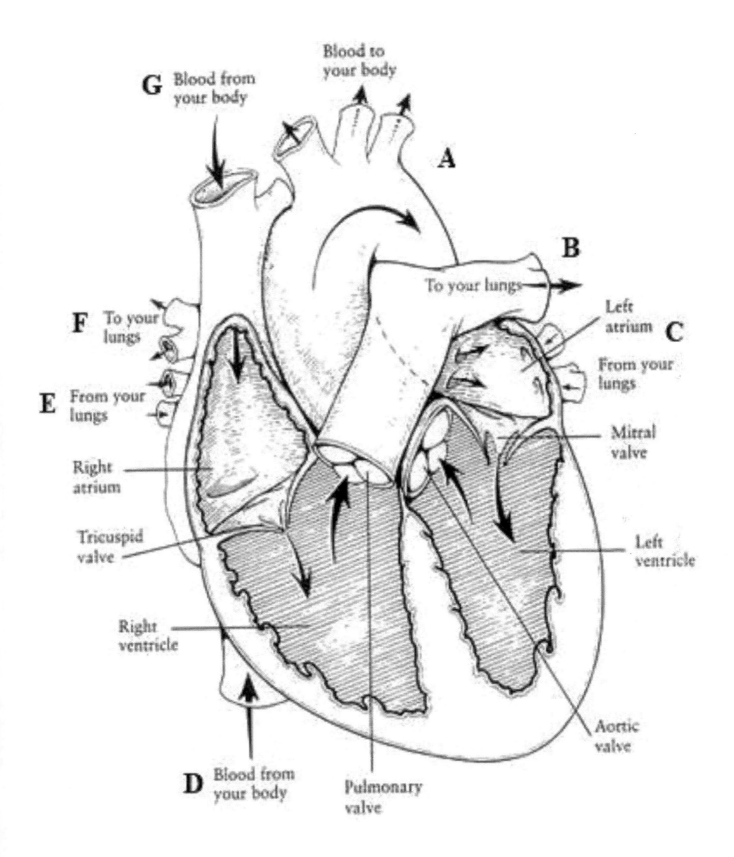

G Blood from your body

Blood to your body

A

B

To your lungs

F To your lungs

E From your lungs

Left atrium

C

From your lungs

Mitral valve

Right atrium

Tricuspid valve

Right ventricle

Left ventricle

D Blood from your body

Pulmonary valve

Aortic valve

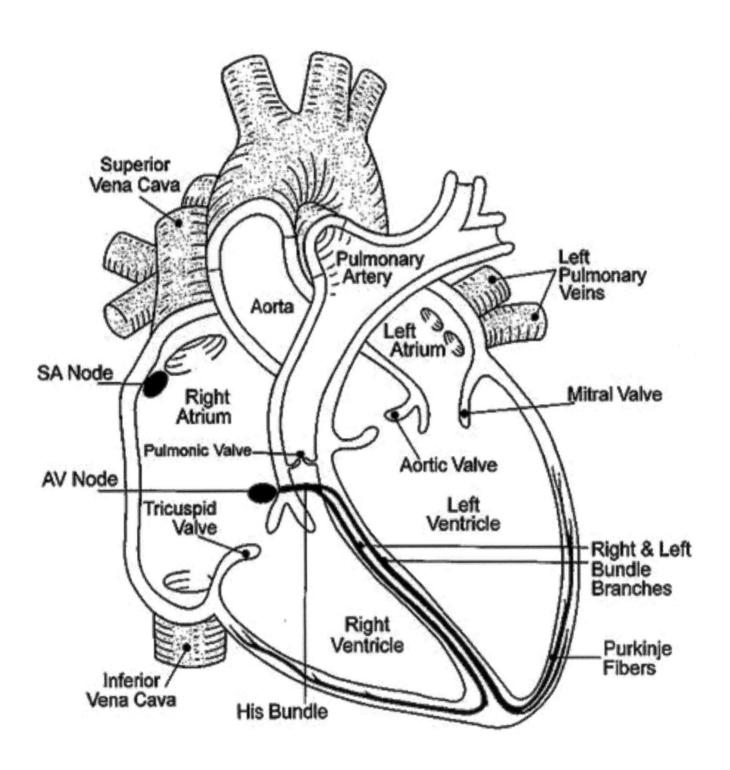

Superior
Vena Cava

Pulmonary
Artery

Aorta

Left
Pulmonary
Veins

Left
Atrium

SA Node

Mitral Valve

Right
Atrium

Pulmonic Valve

AV Node

Aortic Valve

Tricuspid
Valve

Left
Ventricle

Right & Left
Bundle
Branches

Right
Ventricle

Purkinje
Fibers

Inferior
Vena Cava

His Bundle

CARDIOVASCULAR SYSTEM
CHAMBERS OF THE HEART.

CN 17

1. In both drawings, use red for the heavy-lined arrows (representing the flow of oxygenated blood from the lungs) and numbers. Use blue for the light-lined arrows (deoxygenated blood) and numbers. Start the coloring with the superior vena cava (c) and follow the sequence of titles (direction of blood flow.
2. Save bright or dark colors for f, h, i, j, k, l, p.
3. Color in the arrows in the diagram below, starting in the right atrium (1) with blue, and follow the arrows representing blood flow.

SUPERIOR VENA CAVA c
INFERIOR VENA CAVA d

RIGHT ATRIUM i

TRICUSPID VALVE j
CHORDAE TENDINEAE k
PAPILLARY MUSCLE l

RIGHT VENTRICLE m
ENDOCARDIUM h
MYOCARDIUM g
EPICARDIUM
    (VISCERAL PERICARDIUM) f
INTERVENTRICULAR
    SEPTUM g'
PULMONARY SEMILUNAR
    VALVE n

PULMONARY TRUNK b /ARTERY b'
PULMONARY VEINS e

LEFT ATRIUM o

BICUSPID (MITRAL) VALVE p

LEFT VENTRICLE q
AORTIC SEMILUNAR VALVE d

AORTA a

The *heart* is the muscular pump of the blood vascular system—it is the only one in the system. It has four chambers: two on the right relate to the lungs (pulmonary circulation) and two on the left are concerned with the rest of the body (systemic circulation). Deoxygenated blood from the body enters the *right atrium* and is pumped to the lungs by the *right ventricle* under relatively low pressure. Oxygenated blood returns to the *left atrium* and is pumped to the body tissues by the *left ventricle* under rather high pressure, a fact reflected in the thicker left ventricular walls. The *bi-/tricuspid valves* prevent regurgitation of blood back into the atria; the *semilunar valves* prevent reflux of blood back into the ventricles. The *endocardium* is a continuation of the endothelium which lines all blood vessels: simple squamous epithelium. The *myocardium* is cardiac muscle.

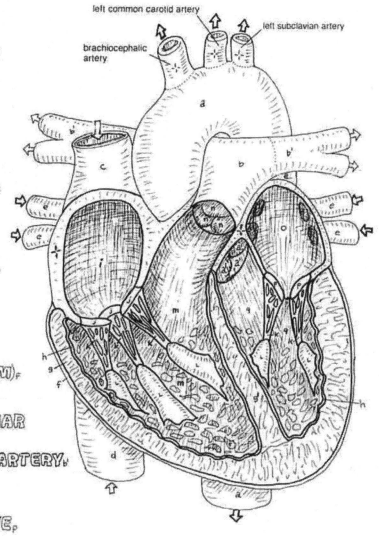

left common carotid artery

left subclavian artery

brachiocephalic artery

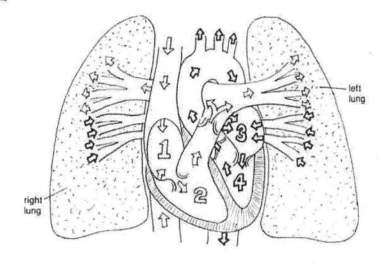

left lung

right lung

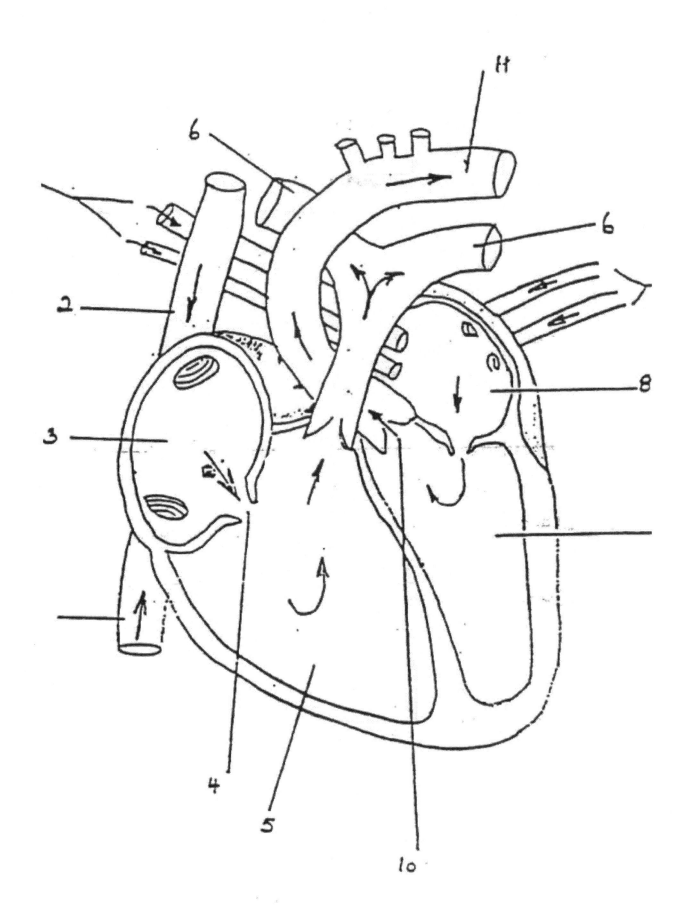

The Heart

blood circulation

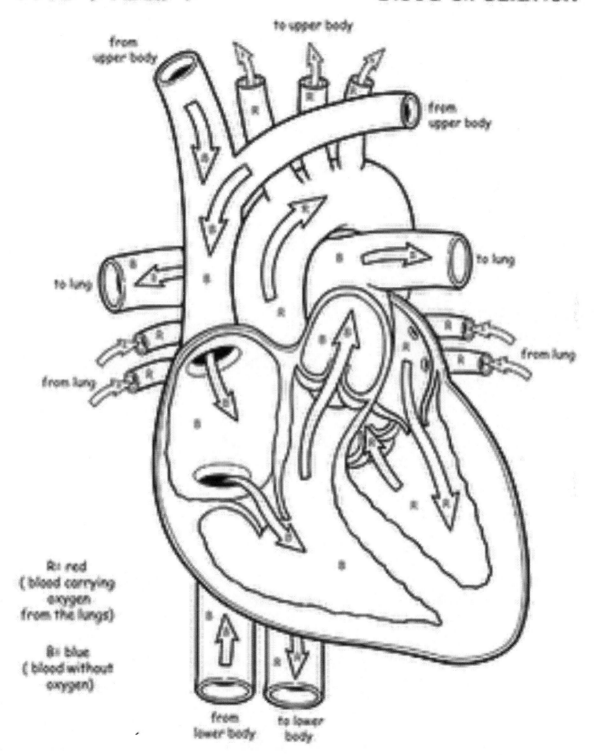

to upper body

from upper body

from upper body

to lung

to lung

from lung

from lung

from lower body

to lower body

R= red
(blood carrying
oxygen
from the lungs)

B= blue
(blood without
oxygen)

The Heart

The heart is a muscular organ that pumps blood to the lungs and to other parts of the body.

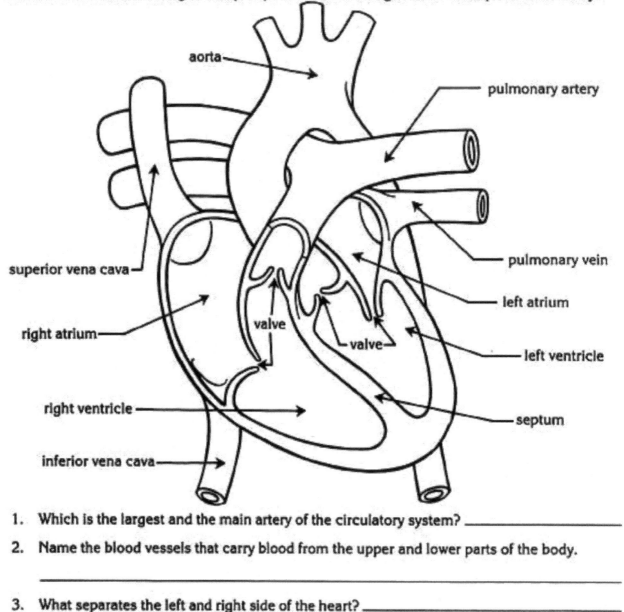

1. Which is the largest and the main artery of the circulatory system? _____

2. Name the blood vessels that carry blood from the upper and lower parts of the body.

   _____

3. What separates the left and right side of the heart? _____

4. Name the blood vessels that carry blood to and from the lungs.

   _____ and _____

5. Name the four chambers of the heart. _____

   _____

6. What keeps blood from flowing back into a chamber of the heart? _____

7. In the diagram of the heart at the top of this page, draw arrows showing the flow of blood through the heart.

Refer to your textbook pages 100-102 to complete the following summary of the Circulatory System.

Purpose and Function of the Circulatory System   *(Fill in the blanks using the terms below.)*

valves   exchange   arteries   veins   contracts   capillaries   oxygen   wastes   nutrients

The function of the circulatory system is to transport _____ and _____ to cells and carry _____ away from cells to the organs responsible for eliminating them from the body.

The heart is a muscular pump. When the heart _____, it produces pressure on the blood in the circulatory system. This pressure pushes blood through the body. The body travels away from the heart in vessels called _____. It returns to the heart through vessels called _____. To stop blood from flowing backwards, flexible flaps of tissue called _____ are found throughout the circulatory system in the heart and veins. Arteries and veins are connected by tiny, thin-walled vessels called _____. These very small vessels are in close contact with the organs and tissues of the body.   The _____ of nutrients, wastes, oxygen and carbon dioxide occur between tissues and the blood through the walls of these small vessels.

Structure of the Heart: Refer to the Diagram on Page 100 to complete the labels of the heart.

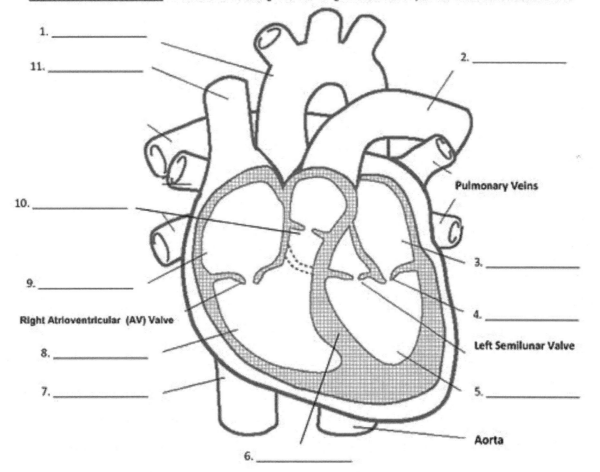

1. _____

11. _____

2. _____

Pulmonary Veins

10. _____

3. _____

9. _____

4. _____

Right Atrioventricular (AV) Valve

Left Semilunar Valve

8. _____

7. _____

5. _____

Aorta

6. _____

Name: _____ Date: _____

Label the identified part of the heart. Color the parts with oxygenated blood in red and deoxygenated blood in purple or deep red. When done complete the chart below with the function and oxygen level of each heart part.

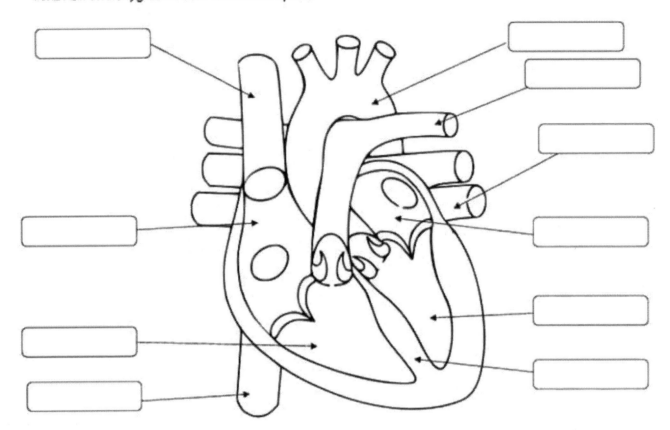

http://commons.wikimedia.org/wiki/File:Heart.svg

	Oxygenated/ Deoxygenated Blood	Function
Vena cava		
Aorta		
Pulmonary Artery		
Pulmonary Vein		
Right Atrium		
Right Ventricle		
Left Atrium		

© 2013 The Tech Savvy Science Teacher http://techsavvyscience.blogspot.com

The Human Heart

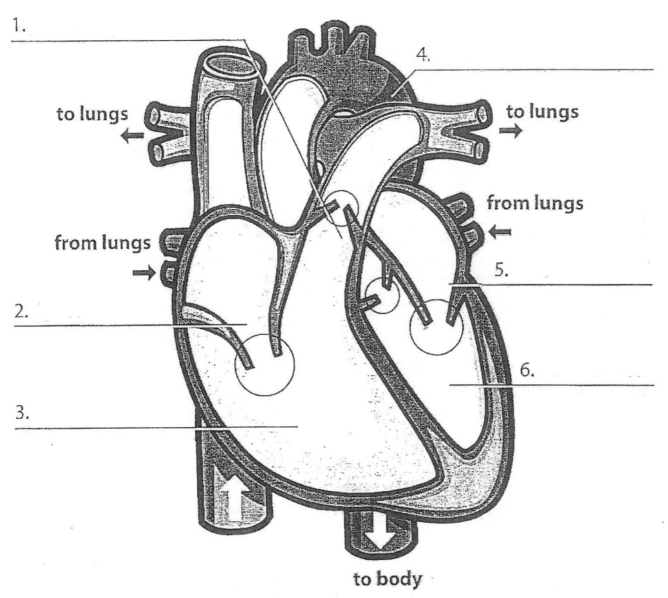

1.

to lungs

4.

to lungs

from lungs

from lungs

2.

5.

3.

6.

to body

WORD BANK

left ventricle	right atrium	pulmonary artery
right ventricle	left atrium	aorta

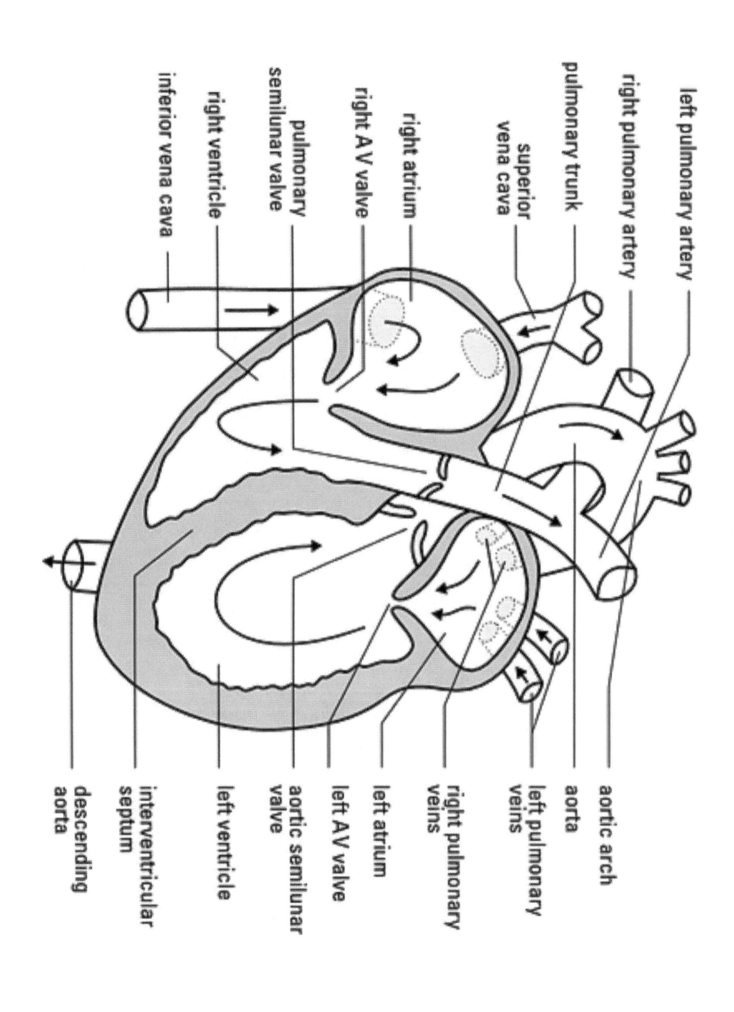

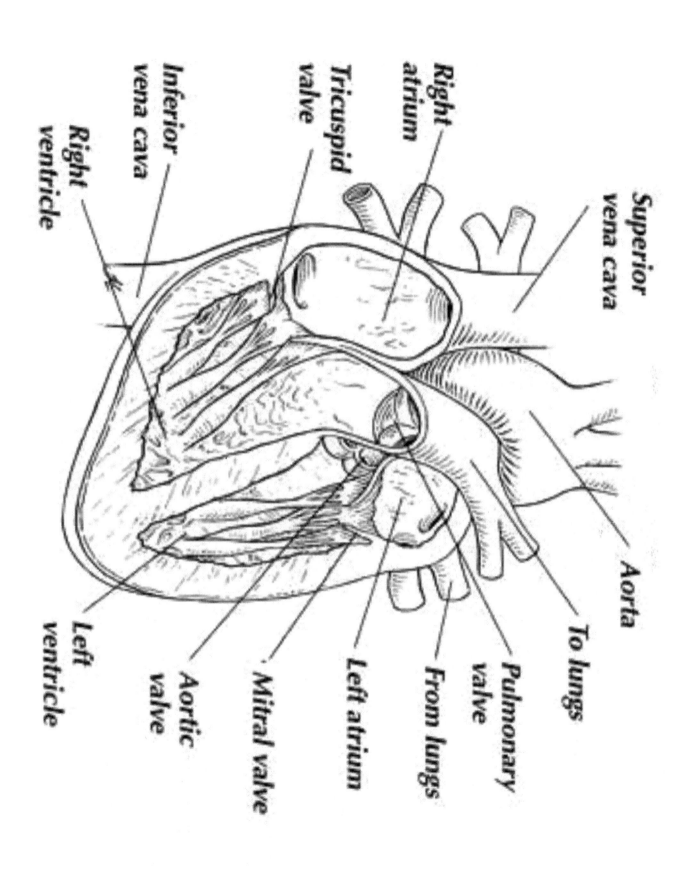

Superior
vena cava

Right
atrium

Tricuspid
valve

Inferior
vena cava

Right
ventricle

Aorta

To lungs

Pulmonary
valve

From lungs

Left atrium

Mitral valve

Aortic
valve

Left
ventricle

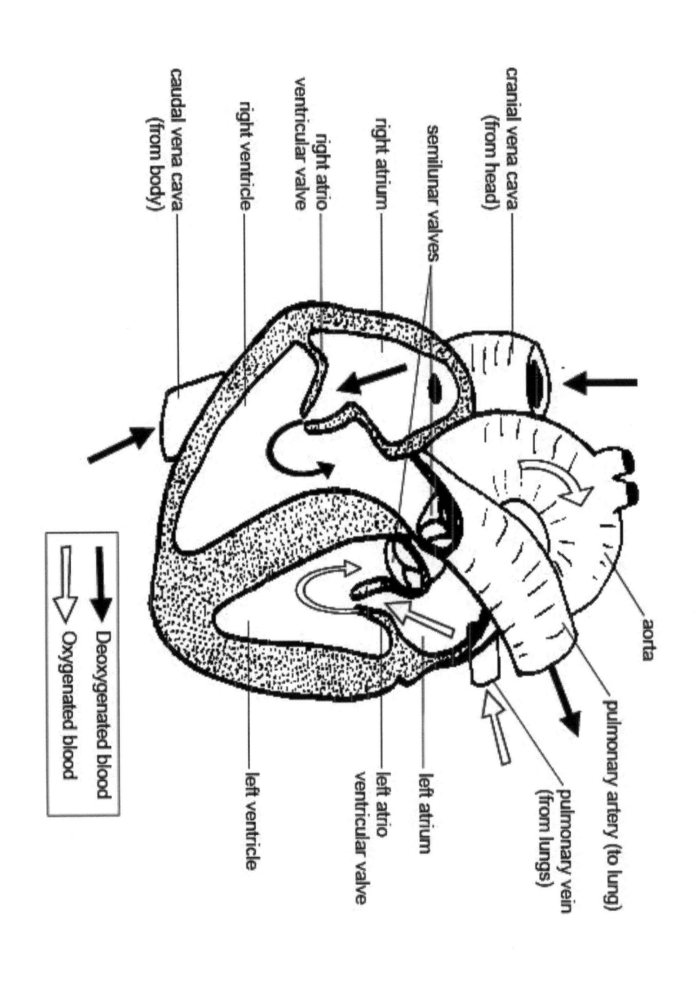

cranial vena cava (from head)

semilunar valves

right atrium

right atrio ventricular valve

right ventricle

caudal vena cava (from body)

aorta

pulmonary artery (to lung)

pulmonary vein (from lungs)

left atrio ventricular valve

left atrium

left ventricle

Deoxygenated blood

Oxygenated blood

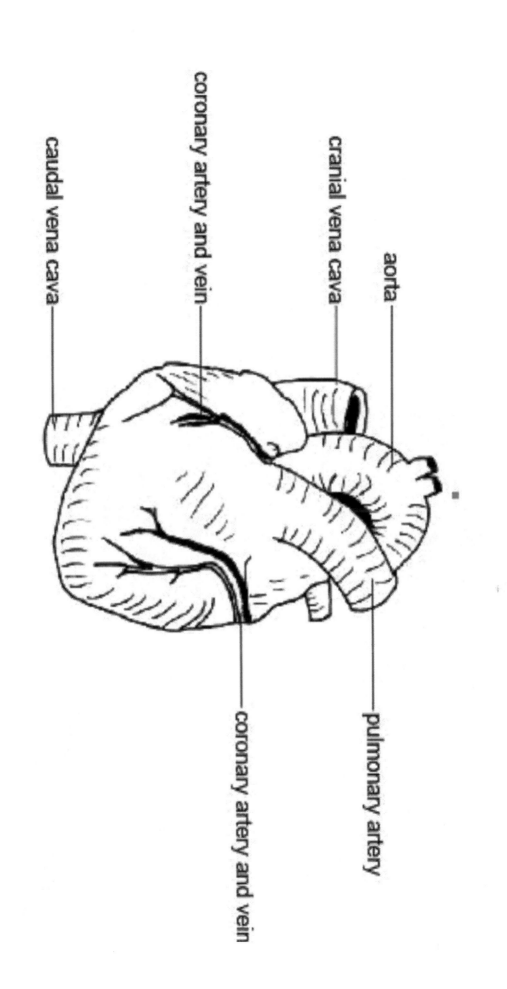

caudal vena cava

coronary artery and vein

cranial vena cava

aorta

coronary artery and vein

pulmonary artery

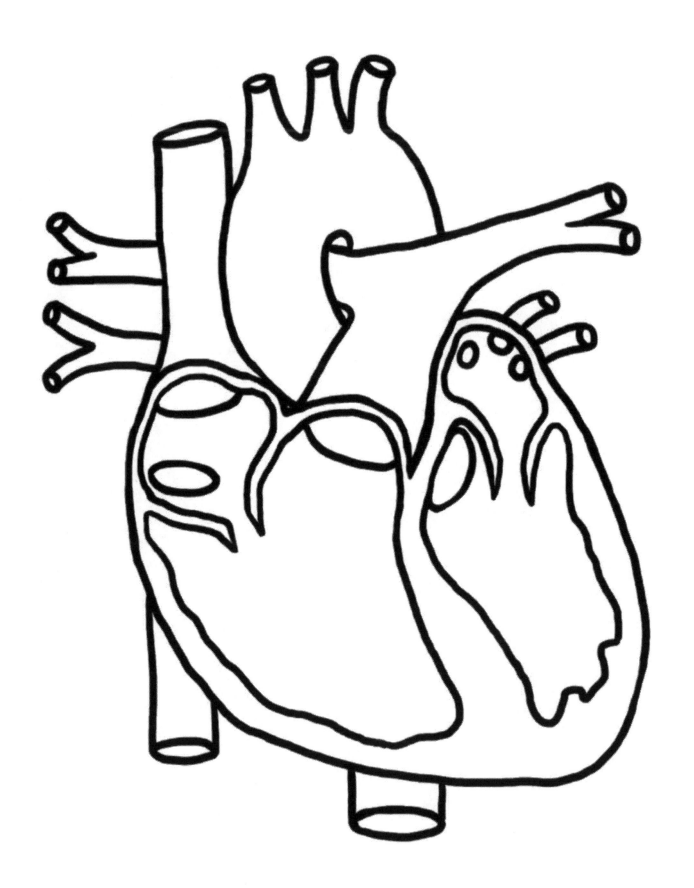

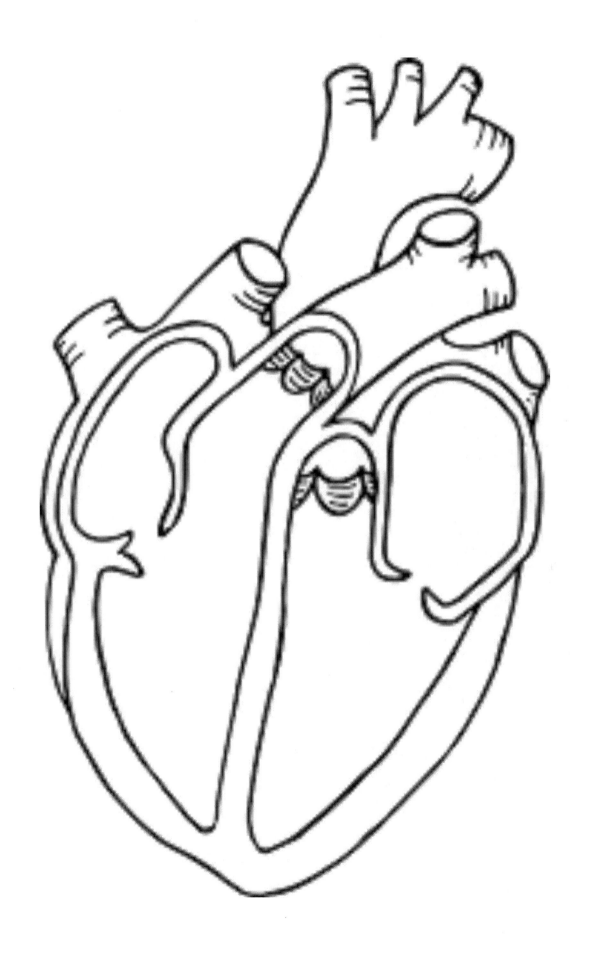

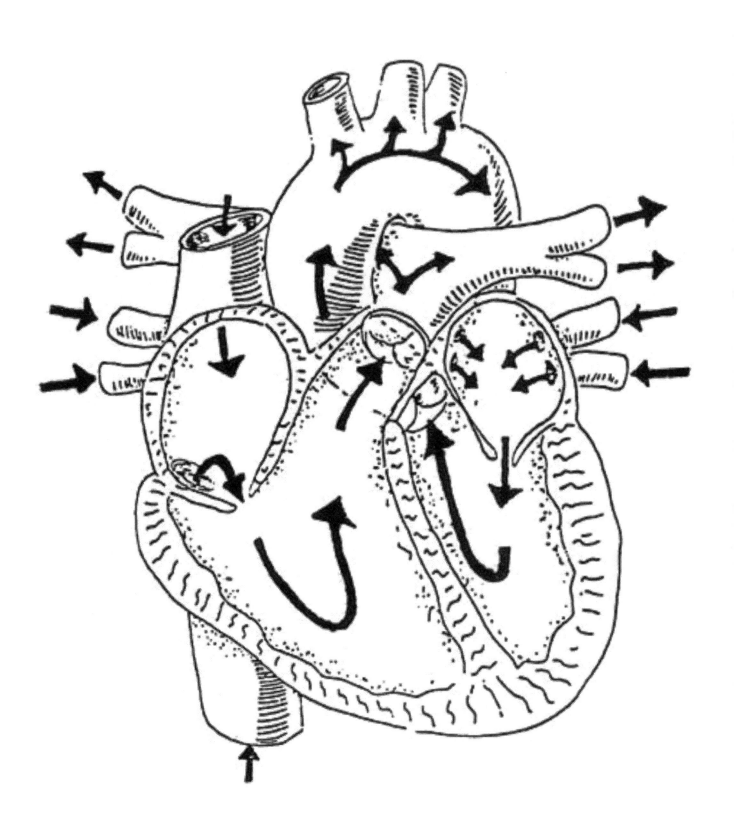

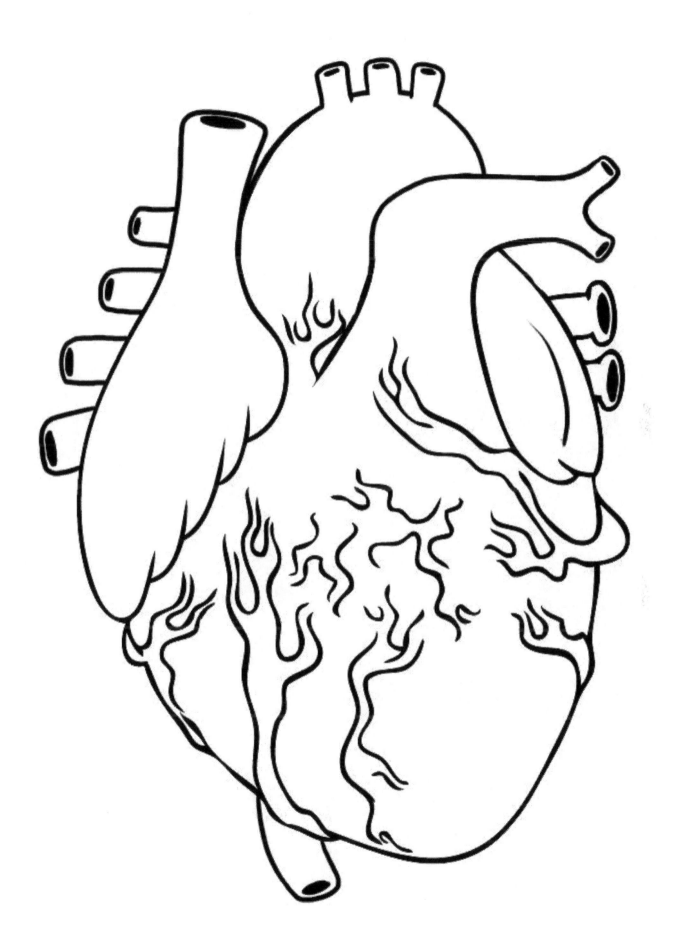

Cardiovascular System

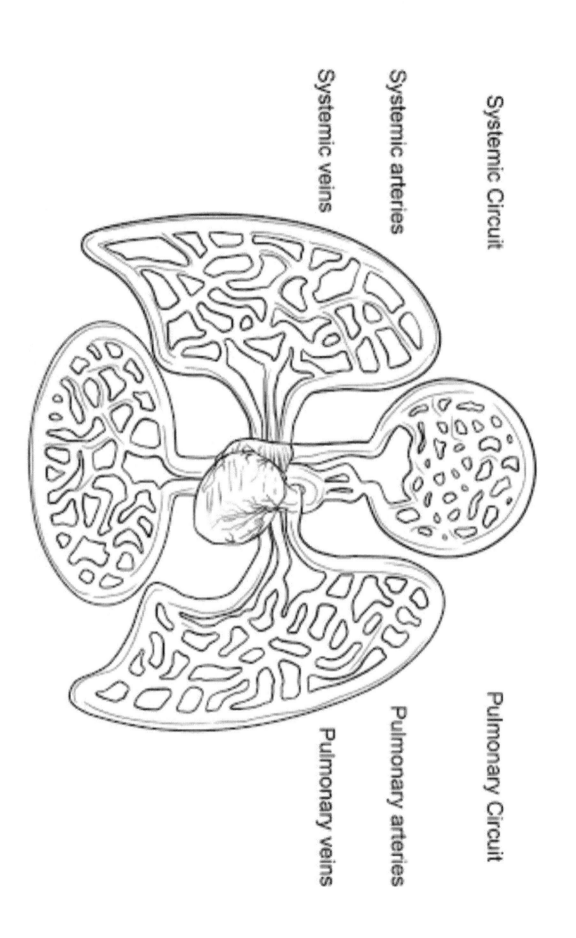

Systemic Circuit

Systemic arteries

Systemic veins

Pulmonary Circuit

Pulmonary arteries

Pulmonary veins

Color the Parts of Pulmonary Circulation

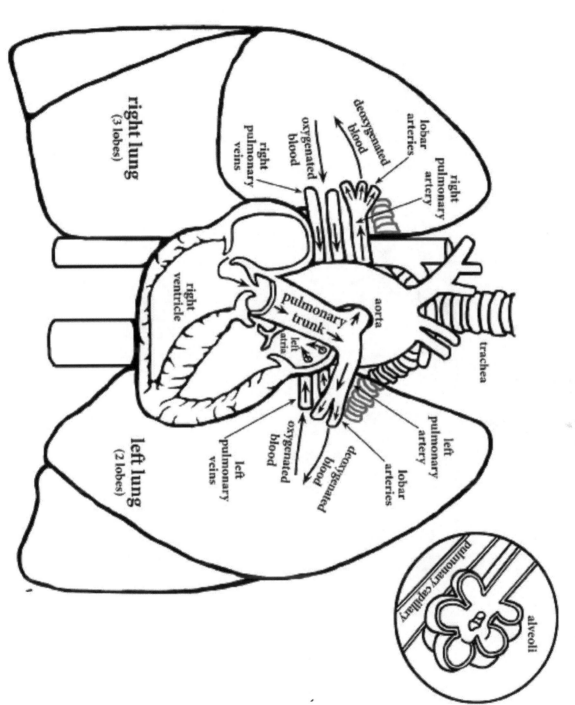

right lung
(3 lobes)

deoxygenated
blood

oxygenated
blood

lobar
arteries

right
pulmonary
veins

right
pulmonary
artery

right
ventricle

pulmonary
trunk

left
atria

aorta

trachea

left
pulmonary
artery

lobar
arteries

deoxygenated
blood

oxygenated
blood

left
pulmonary
veins

left lung
(2 lobes)

pulmonary capillary

alveoli

Pulmonary Circulation

*The heart is made up of four chambers all working together to pump blood around the whole body. The arrows show the blood circulation. The bold arrows represent the flow of **oxygenated** blood. This type of blood flows to all the body parts. It should be colored red. The light arrows represent the flow of **deoxygenated** blood. This type of blood is carried back to the lungs to get oxygen from the air we breathe. It should be colored blue.*

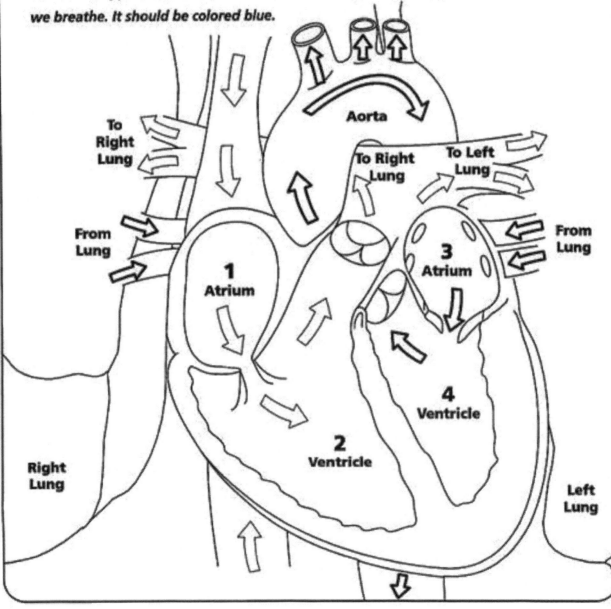

Circulatory System Coloring

PART A

1. Label all parts of the heart.
2. Decide which chambers and vessels carry oxygen-rich blood, and color these RED.
3. Decide which chambers and vessels carry oxygen-poor blood, and color these blue.
4. Describe the pathway of blood as it goes through the heart below in FIVE COMPLETE SENTENCES:

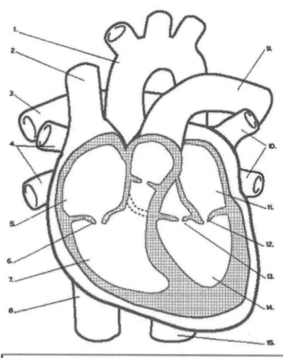

PART B

1. Label all parts of CIRCULATORY SYSTEM SCHEMATIC.
2. Decide which chambers and vessels carry oxygen-rich blood, and color these RED.
3. Decide which chambers and vessels carry oxygen-poor blood, and color these blue.
4. Describe the pathways of pulmonary vs. systemic circulation, and how they are DIFFERENT IN FIVE COMPLETE SENTENCES BELOW.

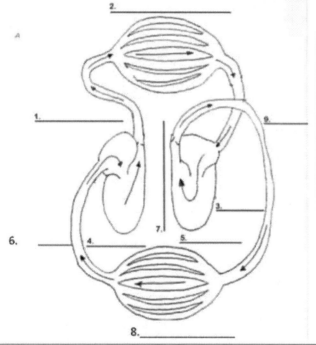

PART C:

Create a graphic organizer below listing the differences between arteries, veins, and capillaries.

Vessels			
Arteries			
Capillaries			
Veins			

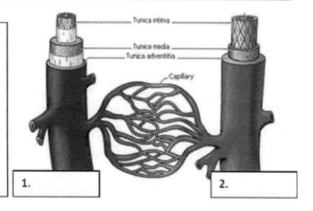

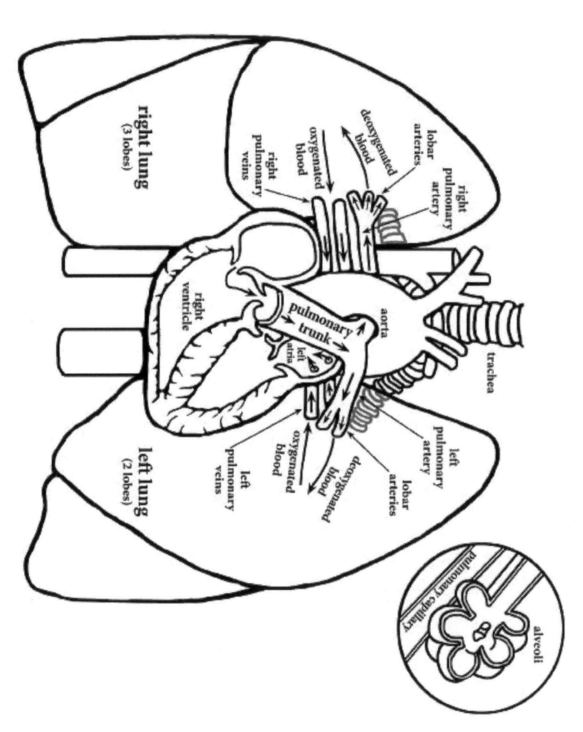

right lung
(3 lobes)

lobar
arteries

deoxygenated
blood

oxygenated
blood

right
pulmonary
veins

right
pulmonary
artery

right
ventricle

pulmonary
trunk

aorta

left
atria

trachea

left
pulmonary
artery

lobar
arteries

deoxygenated
blood

oxygenated
blood

left
pulmonary
veins

left lung
(2 lobes)

pulmonary capillary

alveoli

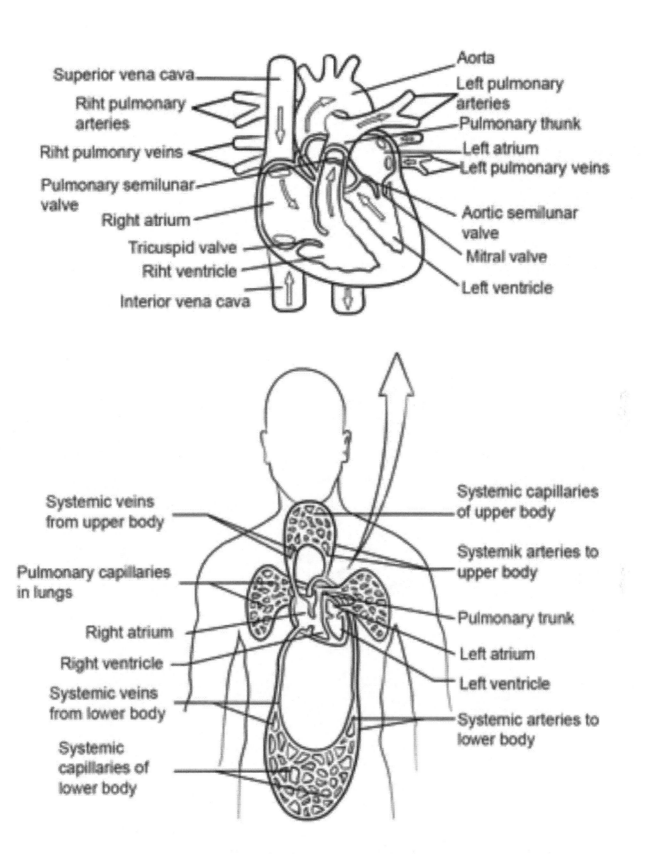

Superior vena cava

Riht pulmonary arteries

Riht pulmonry veins

Pulmonary semilunar valve

Right atrium

Tricuspid valve

Riht ventricle

Interior vena cava

Aorta

Left pulmonary arteries

Pulmonary thunk

Left atrium

Left pulmonary veins

Aortic semilunar valve

Mitral valve

Left ventricle

Systemic veins from upper body

Pulmonary capillaries in lungs

Right atrium

Right ventricle

Systemic veins from lower body

Systemic capillaries of lower body

Systemic capillaries of upper body

Systemik arteries to upper body

Pulmonary trunk

Left atrium

Left ventricle

Systemic arteries to lower body

Human Circulatory System

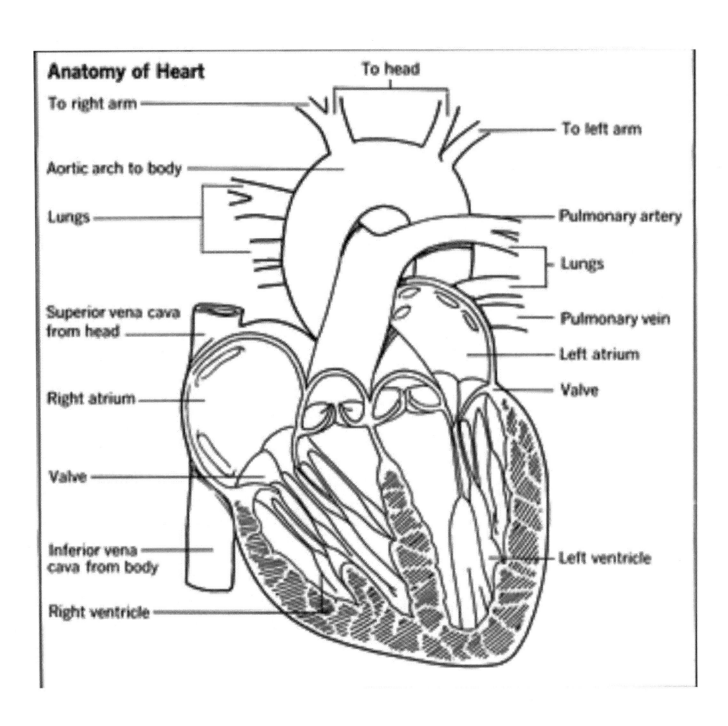

Anatomy of Heart

To right arm

Aortic arch to body

Lungs

Superior vena cava
from head

Right atrium

Valve

Inferior vena
cava from body

Right ventricle

To head

To left arm

Pulmonary artery

Lungs

Pulmonary vein

Left atrium

Valve

Left ventricle

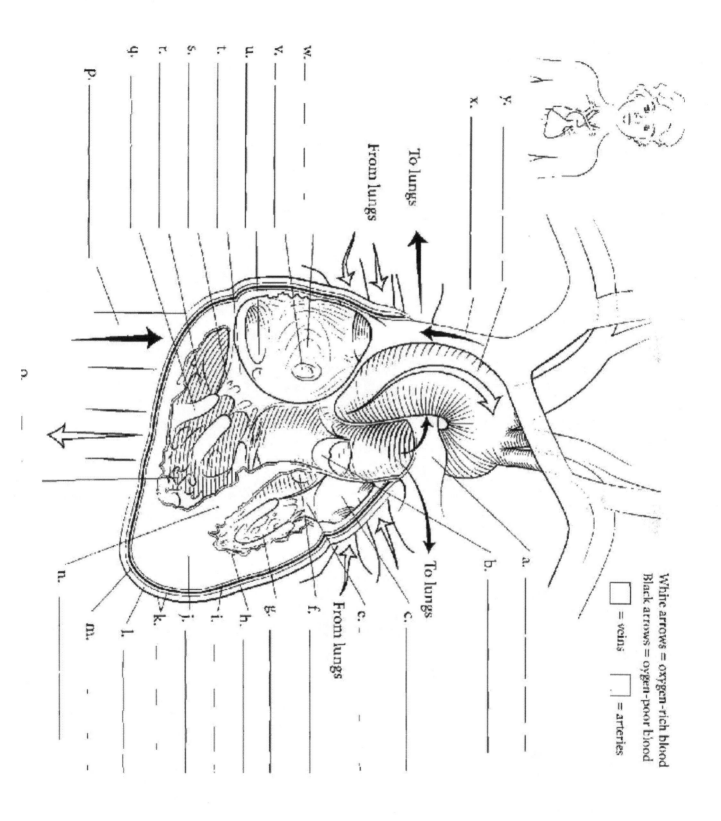

p. ___ ___

q. ___ ___

r. ___ ___

s. ___ ___

t. ___ ___

u. ___ ___

v. ___ ___

w. ___ ___

From lungs

To lungs

y.

x. ___ ___

x. ___ ___

y. ___ ___

a. ___ ___

b. ___ ___

c. ___ ___

c. ___ ___

From lungs

To lungs

d. ___ ___

e. ___ ___

f. ___ ___

g. ___ ___

h. ___ ___

i. ___ ___

j. ___ ___

k. ___ ___

l. ___ ___

m. ___ ___

n. ___ ___

o. ___ ___

White arrows = oxygen-rich blood
Black arrows = oxygen-poor blood

☐ = veins   ☐ = arteries

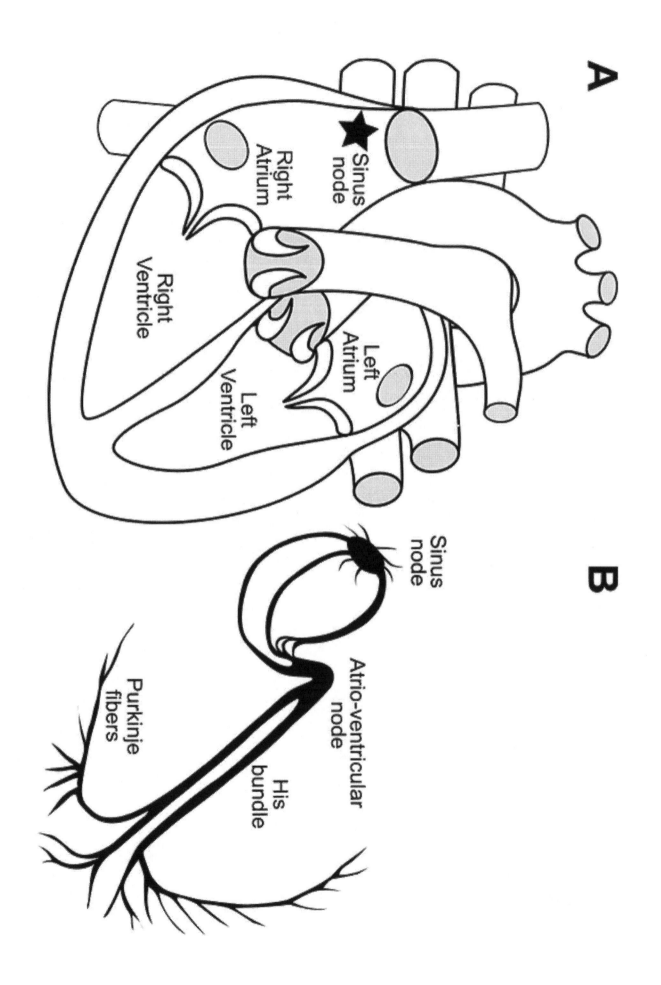

A

Sinus node

Right Atrium

Right Ventricle

Left Atrium

Left Ventricle

B

Sinus node

Atrio-ventricular node

His bundle

Purkinje fibers

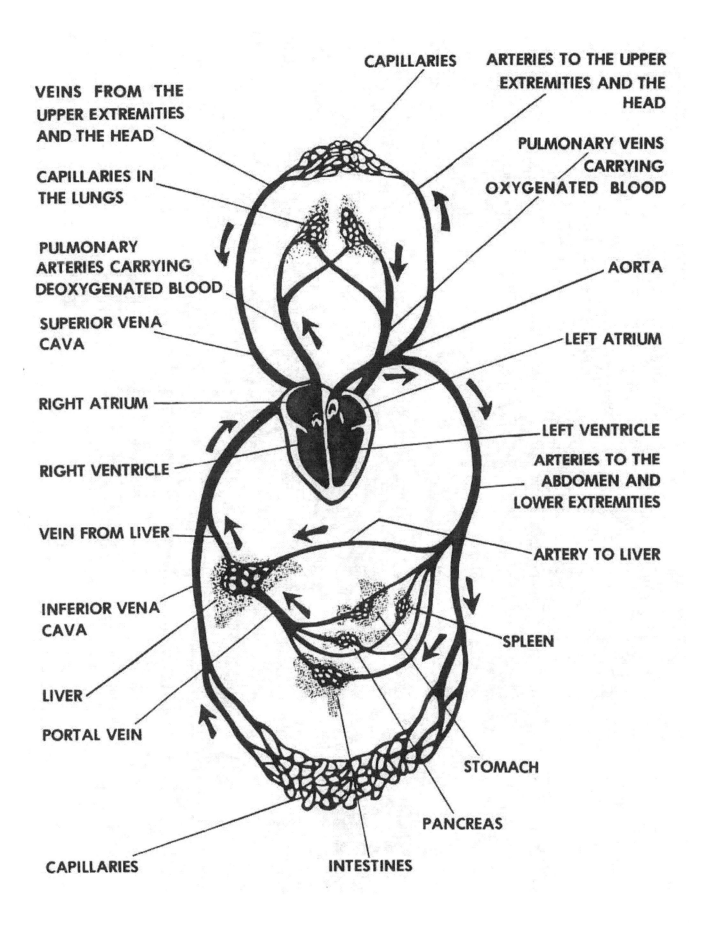

CAPILLARIES

ARTERIES TO THE UPPER EXTREMITIES AND THE HEAD

VEINS FROM THE UPPER EXTREMITIES AND THE HEAD

PULMONARY VEINS CARRYING OXYGENATED BLOOD

CAPILLARIES IN THE LUNGS

PULMONARY ARTERIES CARRYING DEOXYGENATED BLOOD

AORTA

SUPERIOR VENA CAVA

LEFT ATRIUM

RIGHT ATRIUM

LEFT VENTRICLE

ARTERIES TO THE ABDOMEN AND LOWER EXTREMITIES

RIGHT VENTRICLE

VEIN FROM LIVER

ARTERY TO LIVER

INFERIOR VENA CAVA

SPLEEN

LIVER

PORTAL VEIN

STOMACH

CAPILLARIES

PANCREAS

INTESTINES

Cardiovascular Flashcards

Terms on ODD pages and Definitions on EVEN pages

aorta	artery
aortic valve	atrioventricular bundle
arteriole	atrioventricular (AV) node
atrium (p. atria)	atrioventricular valve

a thick-walled blood vessel that, in systemic circulation, carries oxygenated blood away from the heart	largest artery of the body; vessel through which oxygenated blood exits the heart
bundle of fivers in the inter ventricular septum that transfers charges in the heart's conduction system; also called bundle of	valve between the aorta and the left ventricle
specialized part of the interatrial septum that sends a charge to the bundle of His	a tiny artery connecting to a capillary
one of two valves that control blood flow between the atria and ventricles	either of the two upper chambers of the heart

bicuspid valve	blood vessel
blood	bundle of His
blood pressure	capillary
cardiac cycle	carbon dioxide

any of the tubular passageways in the cardiovascular system through which blood travels	atrioventricular valve on the left side of the heart
*see atrioventricular bundle	essential fluid made up of plasma & other elements that circulates throughout the body; delivers nutrients to and removes waste
the smallest blood vessel that forms the exchange point between the arterial and venous vessels	measure of the force of blood surging against the walls of the arteries
waste material transported in the venous blood	repeated contraction and relaxation of the heart as it circulates blood within itself and pumps it out to the rest of the body or the

cardiovascular	coronary artery
carotid artery	depolarization
conduction system	diastole
ductus venosus	ductus arteriousus

blood vessel that supplies oxygen-rich blood to the heart	Relating to or affecting the heart and blood vessels.
contracting state of the myocardial tissue in the heart's conduction system	artery that transports oxygenated blood to the head and neck
relaxation phase of a heartbeat	part of the heart containing specialized tissue that sends electrical charges through heart fibers, causing the heart to
structure in the fetal circulatory system through which blood flows to bypass the fetus's nonfunctioning lungs	structure in the fetal circulatory system through which blood flows to bypass the fetal liver

endocardium	femoral artery
endothelium	foramen ovale
epicardium	heart
left atrium	inferior vena cava

an artery that supplies blood to the thigh	membranous lining of the chambers and valves of the heart; the innermost layer of heart tissue
opening in the septum of the fetal heart that closes at birth	lining of the arteries that secretes substances into the blood
muscular organ that receives blood from the veins and sends it into the arteries	outermost layer of heart tissue
large vein that draws blood from the lower part of the body to the right atrium	upper left heart chamber

left ventricle	myocardium
lumen	pacemaker
mitral valve	pericardium
popliteal artery	polarization

muscular layer of heart tissue between the epicardium and the endocardium	lower left heart chamber
term for the sinoatrial (SA) node; also, an artificial device that regulates heart rhythm	channel inside an artery through which blood flows
protective covering of the heart	*see bicuspid valve
resting state of the myocardial tissue in the conduction system of the heart	an artery that supplies blood to the cells of the area behind the knee

pulmonary artery	pulse
pulmonary valve	repolarization
pulmonary vein	right atrium
saphenous vein	right ventricle

rhythmic expansion and contraction of a blood vessel, usually an artery	one of two arteries that carry blood that is low in oxygen from the heart to the lungs
recharging state; transition from contraction to resting that occurs in the conduction system of the heart	valve that controls the blood flow between the right ventricle and the pulmonary arteries
upper right chamber of the heart	one of four veins that bring oxygenated blood from the lungs to the left atrium
lower right chamber of the heart	any of a group of veins that transport deoxygenated blood from the legs

semilunar valve	sinus rhythm
septum (p. septa)	super vena cava
sinoatrial (SA) node	systole
valve	tricuspid valve

normal heart rhythm	one of the two valves that prevent the back flow of blood flowing out of the heart into the aorta and the pulmonary artery
large vein that transports blood collected from the upper part of the body to the heart	partition between the left and right chambers of the heart
contraction phase of the heartbeat	region of the right atrium containing specialized tissue that sends electrical impulses to the heart muscle, causing it to
atrioventricular valve on the right side of the heart	any of various structures that slow or prevent fluid from flowing backward or forward

vein	venule
vena cava (p. venae cavae)	angiocardiography
ventricle	angiography
arteriography	aortography

a tiny vein connecting to a capillary	any of various blood vessels carrying deoxygenated blood toward the heart, except the pulmonary vein
viewing of the heart and its major blood vessels by x-ray after injection of a contrast medium	*see superior vena cava & inferior vena cava
viewing of the heart's major blood vessels by x-ray after injection of a contrast medium	either of the two lower chambers of the heart
viewing of the aorta by x-ray after injection of a contrast medium	viewing of a specific artery by x-ray after injection of a contrast medium

auscultation	cardiac MRI
cardiac catheterization	cardiac scan
cardiac enzyme tests/studies	cholesterol
doppler ultrasound	digital subtraction angiography

viewing of the heart by magnetic resonance imaging	process of listening to body sounds via a stethoscope
process of viewing the heart muscle at work by scanning the heart of a patient into whom a radioactive substance has been injected	process of passing a thin catheter through an artery or vein to the heart to take blood samples, inject a contrast medium, or
fatty substance present in animal fats; cholesterol circulates int the bloodstream, sometimes causing arterial plaque to form	blood tests for determining levels of enzymes during a myocardial infarction; serum enzyme tests
use of two angiograms done with different dyes to provide a comparison between the results	ultrasound test of blood flow in certain blood vessels

echocardiography	holter monitor
ejection fraction	lipid profile
electrocardiography	multiple-gated acquisition (MUGA) angiography
positron emission tomography (PET) scan	phlebography

portable device that provides a 24-hour electrocardiogram	use of sound waves to produce images showing the structure and motion of the heart
laboratory test that provides the levels of lipids, triglycerides, and other substances in the blood	percentage of the volume of the contents of the left ventricle ejected with each contraction
radioactive scan showing heart function	use of the electrocardiograph in diagnosis
viewing of a vein by x-ray after injection of a contrast medium	type of nuclear image that measures movement of areas of the heart

serum enzyme tests	stress test
sonography	triglyceride
sphygmomanometer	venography
aneurysm	ventriculogram

test that measures heart rate, blood pressure, and other body functions while the patient is exercising on a treadmill	laboratory tests performed to detect enzymes present during or after a myocardial infarction; cardiac enzyme studies
fatty substance; lipid	production of images based on the echoes of sound waves against structures
viewing of a vein by x-ray after injection of a contrast medium	device for measuring blood pressure
x-ray of a ventricle taken after injection of a contrast medium	ballooning of the artery wall caused by weakness in the wall

angina	aortic stenosis
angina pectoris	arrhythmia
aortic regurgitation	arteriosclerosis
asystole	arteritis

narrowing of the aorta	angina pectoris
irregularity in the rhythm of the heartbeat	chest pain, usually caused by a lowered oxygen or blood supply to the heart
hardening of the arteries	backward flow or leakage of blood through a faulty aortic valve
inflammation of an artery or arteries	cardiac arrest

atheroma	atrioventricular block
atherosclerosis	bacterial endocarditis
atrial fibrillation	bradycardia
cardiac arrest	bruit

heart block; partial or complete blockage of the electrical impulses from the atrioventricular node to the ventricles	a fatty deposit (plaque) in the wall of an artery
bacterial inflammation of the inner lining of the heart	hardening of the arteries caused by the buildup of atheromas
heart rate of fewer then 60 beats per minute	an irregular, usually rapid, heartbeat caused by overstimulation of the AV node
sound or murmur, especially an abnormal heart sound heard on auscultation, especially of the carotid artery	sudden stopping of the heart; also called asystole

cardiac tamponade	coarctation of the aorta
cardiomyopathy	congenital heart disease
claudication	constriction
cyanosis	coronary artery disease

abnormal narrowing of the aorta	compression of the heart caused by fluid accumulation in the pericardial sac
heart disease (usually a type of malformation) that exists at birth	disease of the heart muscle
compression or narrowing caused by contraction, as of a vessel	limping caused by inadequate blood supply during activity; usually subsides during rest
condition that reduces the flow of blood and nutrients through the arteries of the heart	bluish or purplish coloration, as of the skin, caused by inadequate oxygenation of the blood

deep vein thrombosis	endocarditis
dysrhythmia	essential hypertension
embolus	fibrillation
gallop	flutter

inflammation of the endocardium, especially an inflammation caused by a bacterial or fungal agent	formation of a thrombus (clot) in a deep vein, such as a femoral vein
high blood pressure without any known cause	abnormal heart rhythm
random, chaotic, irregular heart rhythm	mass of foreign material blocking a vessel
regular but very rapid heartbeat	triple sound of a heartbeat, usually indicative of serious heart disease

heart block	hypertension
hemorrhoid	hypertensive heart disease
high blood pressure	hypotension
infarction	infarct

chronic condition with blood pressure greater than 140/90	*see atrioventricular block
heart disease caused, or worsened, by high blood pressure	varicose condition of veins in the anal region
chronic condition with blood pressure below normal	*see hypertension
area of necrosis caused by a sudden drop in the supply of arterial or venous blood	sudden drop in the supply of arterial or venous blood, often due to an embolus or thrombus

intermittent claudication	low blood pressure
intracardiac tumor	mitral insufficiency / reflux
ischemia	mitral stenosis
murmur	mitral valve prolapse

*see hypotension	attacks of limping, particularly in the legs, due to ischemia of the muscles
backward flow of blood due to a damaged mitral valve	a tumor within one of the heart chambers
abnormal narrowing at the opening of the mitral valve	localized blood insufficiency caused by an obstruction
backward flow of blood into the left atrium due to protrusion of one or both mitral cusps into the left atrium during	soft heart humming sound heard between normal beats

myocardial infarction	occlusion
myocarditis	palpitations
necrosis	patent ductus arteriosus
pericarditits	perfusion deficit

the closing of a blood vessel	sudden drop in the supply of blood to an area of the heart muscle, usually due to a blockage in a coronary artery
uncomfortable pulsations of the heart felt as a thumping in the chest	inflammation of the myocardium
a condition at birth in which the ductus arteriousus, a small duct between the aorta and the pulmonary artery, remains	death of tissue or an organ part due to irreversible damage; usually a result of oxygen deprivation
lack of flow through a blood vessel, usually caused by an occlusion	inflammation of the pericardium

peripheral vascular disease	plaque
petechiae	premature atrial contractions (PACs)
phlebitis	premature ventricular contractions (PVCs)
pulmonary edema	pulmonary artery stenosis

buildup of solid material, such as a fatty deposit, on the lining of an artery	vascular disease in the lower extremities, usually due to the blockages in the arteries of the groin or legs
atrial contractions that occur before the normal impulse; can be the cause of palpitations	minute hemorrhages in the skin
ventricular contractions that occur before the normal impulse; can be the cause of palpitations	inflammation of a vein
narrowing of the pulmonary artery, preventing the lungs from receiving enough blood from the heart to oxygenate	abnormal accumulation of fluid in the lungs

raynaud's phenomenon	rub
rheumatic heart disease	secondary hypertension
risk factor	septal defect
tachycardia	stenosis

frictional sound heard between heartbeats, usually indication a pericardial murmur	spasm in the arteries of the fingers causing numbness or pain
hypertension having a known cause, such as kidney disease	heart valve and/or muscle damage caused by an untreated streptococcal infection
congenital abnormality consisting of an opening in the septum between the atria or ventricles	any of various factors considered to increase the probability that a disease will occur; for example, high blood pressure and smoking
narrowing, particularly of blood vessels or of the cardiac valves	heart rate greater than 100 beats per minute

tetralogy of fallot	thrombotic occlusion
thrombophlebitis	thrombus
thrombosis	tricuspid stenosis
varicose vein	valvulitis

narrowing caused by a thrombus	set of four congenital heart abnormalities appearing together that cause deoxygenated blood to enter the systemic circulation:
stationary blood clot in the cardiovascular system, usually formed from matter found in the blood	inflammation of a vein with a thrombus
abnormal narrowing of the opening of the tricuspid valve	presence of a thrombus in a blood vessel
inflammation of a heart valve	dilated, enlarged, or twisted vein, usually on the leg

vegetation	angioscopy
anastomosis	arteriotomy
angioplasty	atherectomy
balloon valvuloplasty	balloon catheter dilation

viewing of the interior o f a blood vessel using a fiberoptic catheter inserted or threaded into the vessel	clot on a heart valve or opening, usually caused by infection
surgical incision into an artery, especially to remove a clot	surgical connection of two blood vessels to allow blood flow between them
surgical removal of an atheroma	opening of a blocked blood vessel, as by balloon dilation
insertion of a balloon catheter into a blood vessel to open the passage so blood can flow freely	procedure that uses a balloon catheter to open narrowed orifices in cardiac valves

bypass	coronary bypass surgery
cardiopulmonary bypass	embolectomy
coronary angioplasty	endarterectomy
fontan's operation	endovascular surgery

*see bypass	a structure (usually a vein graft) that creates a new passage for blood flow from one artery to another artery or part of an artery;
surgical removal of an embolus	procedure used during surgery to divert blood flow to and from the heart through a heart-lung machine and back into circulation
surgical removal of the diseased portion of the lining of an artery	*see angioplasty
any of various procedures performed during cardiac catheterization, such as angioscopy and atherectomy	surgical procedure that creates a bypass from the right atrium to the main pulmonary artery; fontal's procedure

graft	intravascular stent
heart transplant	percutaneous trans luminal coronary angioplasty
hemorrhoidectomy	phlebotomy
thrombectomy	stent

stent placed within a blood vessel to allow blood to flow freely	any tissue or organ implanted to replace or mend damaged areas
*see balloon catheter dilation	implantation of the heart of a person who has just died into a person whose diseased heart cannot sustain life
drawing blood from a vein via a small incision	surgical removal of hemorrhoids
surgically implanted devices used to hold something (as a blood vessel) open	surgical removal of a thrombus

valve replacement	venipuncture
valvotomy	
valvuloplasty	

small puncture into a vein, usually to draw blood or inject a solution	surgical replacement of a coronary valve
	incision into a cardiac valve to remove an obstruction
	surgical reconstruction of a cardiac valve

Cardiovascular System

Term	Definition
aorta	largest artery of the body; vessel through which oxygenated blood exits the heart
aortic valve	valve between the aorta and the left ventricle
arteriole	a tiny artery connecting to a capillary
artery	a thick-walled blood vessel that, in systemic circulation, carries oxygenated blood away from the heart
atrioventricular bundle	bundle of fivers in the inter ventricular septum that transfers charges in the heart's conduction system; also called bundle of His
atrioventricular (AV) node	specialized part of the interatrial septum that sends a charge to the bundle of His
atrioventricular valve	one of two valves that control blood flow between the atria and ventricles
atrium (p. atria)	either of the two upper chambers of the heart
bicuspid valve	atrioventricular valve on the left side of the heart
blood	essential fluid made up of plasma & other elements that circulates throughout the body; delivers nutrients to and removes waste from the body's cells
blood pressure	measure of the force of blood surging against the walls of the arteries
blood vessel	any of the tubular passageways in the cardiovascular system through which blood travels
bundle of His	*see atrioventricular bundle
capillary	the smallest blood vessel that forms the exchange point between the arterial and venous vessels
carbon dioxide	waste material transported in the venous blood
cardiac cycle	repeated contraction and relaxation of the heart as it circulates blood within itself and pumps it out to the rest of the body or the lungs
cardiovascular	Relating to or affecting the heart and blood vessels.
carotid artery	artery that transports oxygenated blood to the head and neck
conduction system	part of the heart containing specialized tissue that sends electrical charges through heart fibers, causing the heart to contract and relax at regular intervals
coronary artery	blood vessel that supplies oxygen-rich blood to the heart
depolarization	contracting state of the myocardial tissue in the heart's conduction system
diastole	relaxation phase of a heartbeat
ductus arteriousus	structure in the fetal circulatory system through which blood flows to bypass the fetus's nonfunctioning lungs
ductus venosus	structure in the fetal circulatory system through which blood flows to bypass the fetal liver
endocardium	membranous lining of the chambers and valves of the heart; the innermost layer of heart tissue
endothelium	lining of the arteries that secretes substances into the blood
epicardium	outermost layer of heart tissue
femoral artery	an artery that supplies blood to the thigh
foramen ovale	opening in the septum of the fetal heart that closes at birth
heart	muscular organ that receives blood from the veins and sends it into the arteries
inferior vena cava	large vein that draws blood from the lower part of the body to the right atrium
left atrium	upper left heart chamber

left ventricle	lower left heart chamber
lumen	channel inside an artery through which blood flows
mitral valve	*see bicuspid valve
myocardium	muscular layer of heart tissue between the epicardium and the endocardium
pacemaker	term for the sinoatrial (SA) node; also, an artificial device that regulates heart rhythm
pericardium	protective covering of the heart
polarization	resting state of the myocardial tissue in the conduction system of the heart
popliteal artery	an artery that supplies blood to the cells of the area behind the knee
pulmonary artery	one of two arteries that carry blood that is low in oxygen from the heart to the lungs
pulmonary valve	valve that controls the blood flow between the right ventricle and the pulmonary arteries
pulmonary vein	one of four veins that bring oxygenated blood from the lungs to the left atrium
pulse	rhythmic expansion and contraction of a blood vessel, usually an artery
repolarization	recharging state; transition from contraction to resting that occurs in the conduction system of the heart
right atrium	upper right chamber of the heart
right ventricle	lower right chamber of the heart
saphenous vein	any of a group of veins that transport deoxygenated blood from the legs
semilunar valve	one of the two valves that prevent the back flow of blood flowing out of the heart into the aorta and the pulmonary artery
septum (p. septa)	partition between the left and right chambers of the heart
sinoatrial (SA) node	region of the right atrium containing specialized tissue that sends electrical impulses to the heart muscle, causing it to contract
sinus rhythm	normal heart rhythm
super vena cava	large vein that transports blood collected from the upper part of the body to the heart
systole	contraction phase of the heartbeat
tricuspid valve	atrioventricular valve on the right side of the heart
valve	any of various structures that slow or prevent fluid from flowing backward or forward
vein	any of various blood vessels carrying deoxygenated blood toward the heart, except the pulmonary vein
vena cava (p. venae cavae)	*see superior vena cava & inferior vena cava
ventricle	either of the two lower chambers of the heart
venule	a tiny vein connecting to a capillary
angiocardiography	viewing of the heart and its major blood vessels by x-ray after injection of a contrast medium
angiography	viewing of the heart's major blood vessels by x-ray after injection of a contrast medium
aortography	viewing of the aorta by x-ray after injection of a contrast medium
arteriography	viewing of a specific artery by x-ray after injection of a contrast medium
auscultation	process of listening to body sounds via a stethoscope
cardiac catheterization	process of passing a thin catheter through an artery or vein to the heart to take blood samples, inject a contrast medium, or measure various pressures
cardiac enzyme tests/studies	blood tests for determining levels of enzymes during a myocardial infarction; serum enzyme tests
cardiac MRI	viewing of the heart by magnetic resonance imaging
cardiac scan	process of viewing the heart muscle at work by scanning the heart of a patient into

	whom a radioactive substance has been injected
cholesterol	fatty substance present in animal fats; cholesterol circulates int the bloodstre sometimes causing arterial plaque to form
digital subtraction angiography	use of two angiograms done with different dyes to provide a comparison between the results
doppler ultrasound	ultrasound test of blood flow in certain blood vessels
echocardiography	use of sound waves to produce images showing the structure and motion of the heart
ejection fraction	percentage of the volume of the contents of the left ventricle ejected with each contraction
electrocardiography	use of the electrocardiograph in diagnosis
holter monitor	portable device that provides a 24-hour electrocardiogram
lipid profile	laboratory test that provides the levels of lipids, triglycerides, and other substances in the blood
multiple-gated acquisition (MUGA) angiography	radioactive scan showing heart function
phlebography	viewing of a vein by x-ray after injection of a contrast medium
positron emission tomography (PET) scan	type of nuclear image that measures movement of areas of the heart
serum enzyme tests	laboratory tests performed to detect enzymes present during or after a myocardial infarction; cardiac enzyme studies
sonography	production of images based on the echoes of sound waves against structures
sphygmomanometer	device for measuring blood pressure
stress test	test that measures heart rate, blood pressure, and other body functions while the patient is exercising on a treadmill
triglyceride	fatty substance; lipid
venography	viewing of a vein by x-ray after injection of a contrast medium
ventriculogram	x-ray of a ventricle taken after injection of a contrast medium
aneurysm	ballooning of the artery wall caused by weakness in the wall
angina	angina pectoris
angina pectoris	chest pain, usually caused by a lowered oxygen or blood supply to the heart
aortic regurgitation	backward flow or leakage of blood through a faulty aortic valve
aortic stenosis	narrowing of the aorta
arrhythmia	irregularity in the rhythm of the heartbeat
arteriosclerosis	hardening of the arteries
arteritis	inflammation of an artery or arteries
asystole	cardiac arrest
atheroma	a fatty deposit (plaque) in the wall of an artery
atherosclerosis	hardening of the arteries caused by the buildup of atheromas
atrial fibrillation	an irregular, usually rapid, heartbeat caused by overstimulation of the AV node
atrioventricular block	heart block; partial or complete blockage of the electrical impulses from the atrioventricular node to the ventricles
bacterial endocarditis	bacterial inflammation of the inner lining of the heart
bradycardia	heart rate of fewer then 60 beats per minute
bruit	sound or murmur, especially an abnormal heart sound heard on auscultation, especially of the carotid artery
cardiac arrest	sudden stopping of the heart; also called asystole

cardiac tamponade	compression of the heart caused by fluid accumulation in the pericardial sac
cardiomyopathy	disease of the heart muscle
claudication	limping caused by inadequate blood supply during activity; usually subsides during rest
coarctation of the aorta	abnormal narrowing of the aorta
congenital heart disease	heart disease (usually a type of malformation) that exists at birth
constriction	compression or narrowing caused by contraction, as of a vessel
coronary artery disease	condition that reduces the flow of blood and nutrients through the arteries of the heart
cyanosis	bluish or purplish coloration, as of the skin, caused by inadequate oxygenation of the blood
deep vein thrombosis	formation of a thrombus (clot) in a deep vein, such as a femoral vein
dysrhythmia	abnormal heart rhythm
embolus	mass of foreign material blocking a vessel
endocarditis	inflammation of the endocardium, especially an inflammation caused by a bacterial or fungal agent
essential hypertension	high blood pressure without any known cause
fibrillation	random, chaotic, irregular heart rhythm
flutter	regular but very rapid heartbeat
gallop	triple sound of a heartbeat, usually indicative of serious heart disease
heart block	*see atrioventricular block
hemorrhoid	varicose condition of veins in the anal region
high blood pressure	*see hypertension
hypertension	chronic condition with blood pressure greater than 140/90
hypertensive heart disease	heart disease caused, or worsened, by high blood pressure
hypotension	chronic condition with blood pressure below normal
infarct	area of necrosis caused by a sudden drop in the supply of arterial or venous blood
infarction	sudden drop in the supply of arterial or venous blood, often due to an embolus or thrombus
intermittent claudication	attacks of limping, particularly in the legs, due to ischemia of the muscles
intracardiac tumor	a tumor within one of the heart chambers
ischemia	localized blood insufficiency caused by an obstruction
low blood pressure	*see hypotension
mitral insufficiency / reflux	backward flow of blood due to a damaged mitral valve
mitral stenosis	abnormal narrowing at the opening of the mitral valve
mitral valve prolapse	backward flow of blood into the left atrium due to protrusion of one or both mitral cusps into the left atrium during contractions
murmur	soft heart humming sound heard between normal beats
myocardial infarction	sudden drop in the supply of blood to an area of the heart muscle, usually due to a blockage in a coronary artery
myocarditis	inflammation of the myocardium
necrosis	death of tissue or an organ part due to irreversible damage; usually a result of oxygen deprivation

occlusion	the closing of a blood vessel
palpitations	uncomfortable pulsations of the heart felt as a thumping in the chest
patent ductus arteriosus	a condition at birth in which the ductus arteriousus, a small duct between the aorta and the pulmonary artery, remains abnormally open
perfusion deficit	lack of flow through a blood vessel, usually caused by an occlusion
pericarditits	inflammation of the pericardium
peripheral vascular disease	vascular disease in the lower extremities, usually due to the blockages in the arteries of the groin or legs
petechiae	minute hemorrhages in the skin
phlebitis	inflammation of a vein
plaque	buildup of solid material, such as a fatty deposit, on the lining of an artery
premature atrial contractions (PACs)	atrial contractions that occur before the normal impulse; can be the cause of palpitations
premature ventricular contractions (PVCs)	ventricular contractions that occur before the normal impulse; can be the cause of palpitations
pulmonary artery stenosis	narrowing of the pulmonary artery, preventing the lungs from receiving enough blood from the heart to oxygenate
pulmonary edema	abnormal accumulation of fluid in the lungs
raynaud's phenomenon	spasm in the arteries of the fingers causing numbness or pain
rheumatic heart disease	heart valve and/or muscle damage caused by an untreated streptococcal infection
risk factor	any of various factors considered to increase the probability that a disease will occur; for example, high blood pressure and smoking are considered risk factors for heart disease
rub	frictional sound heard between heartbeats, usually indication a pericardial murmur
secondary hypertension	hypertension having a known cause, such as kidney disease
septal defect	congenital abnormality consisting of an opening in the septum between the atria or ventricles
stenosis	narrowing, particularly of blood vessels or of the cardiac valves
tachycardia	heart rate greater than 100 beats per minute
tetralogy of fallot	set of four congenital heart abnormalities appearing together that cause deoxygenated blood to enter the systemic circulation: ventricular septal defect, pulmonary stenosis, incorrect position of the aorta, and rich ventricular hypertrophy
thrombophlebitis	inflammation of a vein with a thrombus
thrombosis	presence of a thrombus in a blood vessel
thrombotic occlusion	narrowing caused by a thrombus
thrombus	stationary blood clot in the cardiovascular system, usually formed from matter found in the blood
tricuspid stenosis	abnormal narrowing of the opening of the tricuspid valve
valvulitis	inflammation of a heart valve
varicose vein	dilated, enlarged, or twisted vein, usually on the leg
vegetation	clot on a heart valve or opening, usually caused by infection
anastomosis	surgical connection of two blood vessels to allow blood flow between them
angioplasty	opening of a blocked blood vessel, as by balloon dilation
angioscopy	viewing of the interior o f a blood vessel using a fiberoptic catheter inserted or threaded into the vessel

arteriotomy	surgical incision into an artery, especially to remove a clot
atherectomy	surgical removal of an atheroma
balloon catheter dilation	insertion of a balloon catheter into a blood vessel to open the passage so blood can flow freely
balloon valvuloplasty	procedure that uses a balloon catheter to open narrowed orifices in cardiac valves
bypass	a structure (usually a vein graft) that creates a new passage for blood flow from one artery to another artery or part of an artery; used to create a detour around blockages in the arteries
cardiopulmonary bypass	procedure used during surgery to divert blood flow to and from the heart through a heart-lung machine and back into circulation
coronary angioplasty	*see angioplasty
coronary bypass surgery	*see bypass
embolectomy	surgical removal of an embolus
endarterectomy	surgical removal of the diseased portion of the lining of an artery
endovascular surgery	any of various procedures performed during cardiac catheterization, such as angioscopy and atherectomy
fontan's operation	surgical procedure that creates a bypass from the right atrium to the main pulmonary artery; fontal's procedure
graft	any tissue or organ implanted to replace or mend damaged areas
heart transplant	implantation of the heart of a person who has just died into a person whose diseased heart cannot sustain life
hemorrhoidectomy	surgical removal of hemorrhoids
intravascular stent	stent placed within a blood vessel to allow blood to flow freely
percutaneous trans luminal coronary angioplasty	*see balloon catheter dilation
phlebotomy	drawing blood from a vein via a small incision
stent	surgically implanted devices used to hold something (as a blood vessel) open
thrombectomy	surgical removal of a thrombus
valve replacement	surgical replacement of a coronary valve
valvotomy	incision into a cardiac valve to remove an obstruction
valvuloplasty	surgical reconstruction of a cardiac valve
venipuncture	small puncture into a vein, usually to draw blood or inject a solution

Cardiovascular
Flashcard Activity

Terminology #6 Word Search Puzzle

```
C T I S O P E D A M A G E N O I T I D N O C I M P U L S E E V E C X E
F A Z T G X A I E T R S E L Y T U O H G U O R H T R O F Q N N U M S S
X S U K I S S L Z S L F T W L Y R B S P L D E T A N E G Y X O U T P P
J L E S U S C S S E A V U M L L L E J E R C I P S F S S Z T I H X E E
W O A I E I S Y S R I P N Y A X T T S N T O A M V X U C S R Y Y E C C
Z M D R R D B U R R E I I G U L A S B O S H V A P N P T T U I N X I I
B E U T O E G Y E A E B M H S G E O G I W N R I X U P A A K R F I A A
E Q N I L M T B P C N B M P U V B M I T K I L E D Q L P J Y O E P L L
I E N D R T E R I A E O M A E L T R U C O M A X K E Y S N P V U G I L
V T D A A T S F A I S O M A H I R E W U C I T R O A S O E B P P X Z Y
H B R P W Y A S J D W S A L H C A N S D L I P M R G G N N E E W T E B
J C Q E L D N U B R A Z U A U C E N B N B Y E B N O I T I D N O C D M
N C E T N E M E C A L P E R L P H I D O E O S W Y N N O I T R O P S X
H N D X R N O I T C E J N I G P P T W C D L A Q G K I Z U Y N C Y Z S
O X Y G E N A T E D I S E A S E M H T Y H R T R A E H L A M R O N T O
```

☐TISSUE   ☐PRESSURE   ☐VENTRICLE
☐ARTERIES   ☐CARDIAC ARREST   ☐CAUSED
☐SUPPLY   ☐DISEASE   ☐AORTIC
☐PROVIDES   ☐VESSEL   ☐OPENING
☐CHAMBERS   ☐DEPOSIT   ☐BETWEEN
☐NORMAL HEART RHYTHM ☐PULMONARY   ☐BETWEEN
☐USUALLY   ☐CONDUCTION   ☐SPECIALIZED
☐HEARTBEAT   ☐INNERMOST   ☐IMPULSE
☐DAMAGE   ☐FEMORAL   ☐SEPTAL
☐MINUTE   ☐INJECTION   ☐BYPASS
☐THROUGHOUT   ☐REPLACEMENT   ☐CONDITION
☐CHAMBERS   ☐BUNDLE   ☐VARIOUS
☐ATRIUM   ☐OXYGENATED   ☐OXYGENATED
☐CONDITION   ☐ESPECIALLY   ☐ATRIUM
☐IMPULSE   ☐PORTION

Terminology #6 Word Search Puzzle

```
K C T R W A T X S H D J L D A O C X A A P J B E S N T A F N R V A B P
N G A E O Q Y D R A E U J M Z D A Q K R E Y U H C W O I N C I Q E L H
M G W R V R K P Y Z P A C K S B R T Y J T I F Y V R W D O J G Y V O L
U N T D O L I Q O C K H R T B J D S R V E E O N T X G H I T H V L O E
S A K R B T A G O C D P E T U M I K I P C Z R I B M I E T P T E A D B
G K M M T T I V H J S N M N O S O C U T H Q C I A H T A A S V G V V I
Y E R X V S L D V T T O N D O W V G I A I V S M T S A R T I E E R E T
P U L S E A Y K A A A L I K T U A E P S A L O H U I G T L S N T A S S
T A I M H T Y H R R A T X G C A S A N L E R U L L O S B U O T A N S Y
C O R O N A R Y A R T F R Y N H C V V O E G O V I V V L C N R T U E Y
S O N O G R A P H Y E E H I J A U E E H S B W G L S R O S A I I L L R
E A I D R A C Y D A R B R S U X L Y T I M U N F M A Z C U Y C O I D E
F Y T S A L P O I G N A V Y A M A A R E N A S D E O V K A C L N M S T
E L O R E T S E L O H C R W T H R O M B U S O H B L U M E N E O E O R
C L A J D R O M U T C A I D R A C A R T N I V E N O G R A P H Y S W A
```

☐CORONARY ARTERY ☐ANGIOGRAPHY ☐ANGIOSCOPY
☐CARDIOVASCULAR ☐PETECHIAE ☐AORTIC VALVE
☐RIGHT VENTRICLE ☐INTRACARDIAC TUMOR ☐DUCTUS VENOSUS
☐CAROTID ARTERY ☐AUSCULTATION ☐LUMEN
☐THROMBUS ☐PULSE ☐VEGETATION
☐SEMILUNAR VALVE ☐BLOOD VESSEL ☐PHLEBITIS
☐VENOGRAPHY ☐SONOGRAPHY ☐CYANOSIS
☐VALVE ☐ARRHYTHMIA ☐RIGHT ATRIUM
☐ARTERY ☐ATHEROMA ☐EMBOLUS
☐ARTERITIS ☐BRADYCARDIA ☐ANGIOPLASTY
☐HEART ☐CHOLESTEROL ☐SAPHENOUS VEIN
☐AORTA ☐STENT ☐VALVULITIS
☐HEART BLOCK

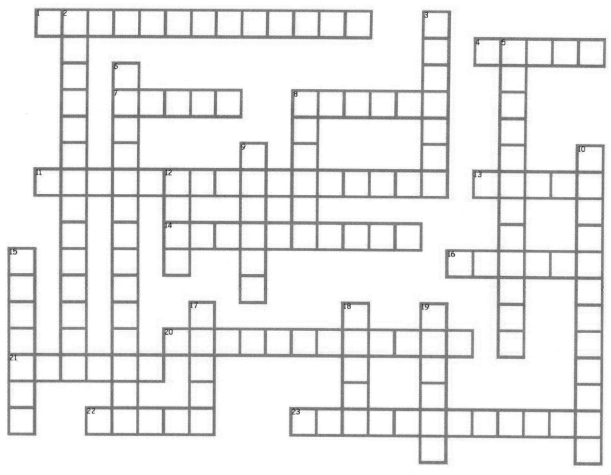

Across

1 laboratory test that provides the levels of lipids, ____, and other substances in the blood
4 any of various structures that slow or prevent fluid from flowing backward or forward
7 largest artery of the body; vessel through which oxygenated blood exits the heart
8 cardiac ____
11 *see ____ block
13 rhythmic expansion and contraction of a blood vessel, usually an artery
14 triple sound of a heartbeat, usually ____ of serious heart disease
16 ballooning of the ____ wall caused by weakness in the wall
20 cardiac enzyme ____
21 *see atrioventricular ____
22 any tissue or organ implanted to replace or mend damaged areas
23 small puncture into a vein, usually to draw blood or inject a solution

Down

2 surgical ____ of a cardiac valve
3 regular but very rapid heartbeat
5 abnormal ____ of fluid in the lungs
6 any of the tubular passageways in the ____ system through which blood travels
8 angina pectoris
9 backward flow of blood into the left atrium due to protrusion of one or both mitral cusps into the left ____ during contractions
10 any of a group of veins that transport ____ blood from the legs
12 any of various blood vessels carrying deoxygenated blood toward the heart, except the pulmonary vein
15 upper right ____ of the heart
17 muscular organ that receives blood from the veins and sends it into the arteries
18 channel inside an artery through which blood flows
19 bundle of fivers in the inter ventricular ____ that transfers charges in the heart's conduction system; also called bundle of His

Terminology #6 Matching

Write the code corresponding to the correct match in the space provided.

____ 1. raynaud's phenomenon

____ 2. depolarization

____ 3. cardiomyopathy

____ 4. capillary

____ 5. atrioventricular block

____ 6. endocarditis

____ 7. angiography

____ 8. venipuncture

____ 9. cardiac catheterization

____ 10. endarterectomy

____ 11. heart block

____ 12. constriction

____ 13. hypertension

____ 14. cardiovascular

____ 15. sphygmomanometer

____ 16. aortic regurgitation

____ 17. pulmonary artery stenosis

____ 18. saphenous vein

____ 19. tachycardia

____ 20. asystole

____ 21. atrioventricular valve

____ 22. hemorrhoidectomy

____ 23. balloon valvuloplasty

____ 24. hemorrhoid

____ 25. ventriculogram

____ 26. mitral stenosis

____ 27. semilunar valve

____ 28. arrhythmia

____ 29. systole

____ 30. atherosclerosis

____ 31. coronary artery disease

A1. abnormal narrowing at the opening of the mitral valve

B1. an artery that supplies blood to the cells of the area behind the knee

C1. chronic condition with blood pressure greater than 140/90

D1. atrioventricular valve on the left side of the heart

E1. ultrasound test of blood flow in certain blood vessels

F1. surgical removal of the diseased portion of the lining of an artery

G1. surgical removal of an atheroma

H1. valve that controls the blood flow between the right ventricle and the pulmonary arteries

I1. implantation of the heart of a person who has just died into a person whose diseased heart cannot sustain life

J1. random, chaotic, irregular heart rhythm

K1. sudden drop in the supply of arterial or venous blood, often due to an embolus or thrombus

L1. dilated, enlarged, or twisted vein, usually on the leg

M1. surgical connection of two blood vessels to allow blood flow between them

N1. large vein that draws blood from the lower part of the body to the right atrium

O1. inflammation of a vein with a thrombus

P1. surgically implanted devices used to hold something (as a blood vessel) open

Q1. irregularity in the rhythm of the heartbeat

R1. one of two valves that control blood flow between the atria and ventricles

S1. relaxation phase of a heartbeat

T1. blood tests for determining levels of enzymes during a myocardial infarction; serum enzyme tests

U1. upper left heart chamber

V1. disease of the heart muscle

W1. cardiac arrest

X1. viewing of the heart and its major blood vessels by x-ray after injection of a contrast medium

Y1. hardening of the arteries caused by the buildup of atheromas

Z1. x-ray of a ventricle taken after injection of a contrast medium

A2. presence of a thrombus in a blood vessel

B2. lining of the arteries that secretes substances into the blood

C2. *see atrioventricular bundle

____ 32. carbon dioxide

____ 33. myocardium

____ 34. pulmonary vein

____ 35. blood pressure

____ 36. aneurysm

____ 37. doppler ultrasound

____ 38. arteriography

____ 39. atrioventricular bundle

____ 40. diastole

____ 41. deep vein thrombosis

____ 42. fontan's operation

____ 43. intermittent claudication

____ 44. intravascular stent

____ 45. tricuspid valve

____ 46. premature atrial contractions (PACs)

____ 47. arteriotomy

____ 48. repolarization

____ 49. arteritis

____ 50. femoral artery

____ 51. necrosis

____ 52. sinoatrial (SA) node

____ 53. vegetation

____ 54. coronary angioplasty

____ 55. cardiac arrest

____ 56. ejection fraction

____ 57. sonography

____ 58. septal defect

____ 59. dysrhythmia

____ 60. risk factor

____ 61. angiocardiography

____ 62. angina pectoris

____ 63. pulmonary edema

____ 64. holter monitor

____ 65. bundle of His

____ 66. tricuspid stenosis

____ 67. ductus arteriousus

____ 68. phlebitis

D2. bluish or purplish coloration, as of the skin, caused by inadequate oxygenation of the blood

E2. inflammation of the endocardium, especially an inflammation caused by a bacterial or fungal agent

F2. normal heart rhythm

G2. *see hypertension

H2. area of necrosis caused by a sudden drop in the supply of arterial or venous blood

I2. heart valve and/or muscle damage caused by an untreated streptococcal infection

J2. one of two arteries that carry blood that is low in oxygen from the heart to the lungs

K2. clot on a heart valve or opening, usually caused by infection

L2. chronic condition with blood pressure below normal

M2. viewing of the aorta by x-ray after injection of a contrast medium

N2. use of two angiograms done with different dyes to provide a comparison between the results

O2. laboratory test that provides the levels of lipids, triglycerides, and other substances in the blood

P2. an artery that supplies blood to the thigh

Q2. limping caused by inadequate blood supply during activity; usually subsides during rest

R2. heart disease caused, or worsened, by high blood pressure

S2. sudden stopping of the heart; also called asystole

T2. type of nuclear image that measures movement of areas of the heart

U2. stent placed within a blood vessel to allow blood to flow freely

V2. process of listening to body sounds via a stethoscope

W2. high blood pressure without any known cause

X2. largest artery of the body; vessel through which oxygenated blood exits the heart

Y2. backward flow of blood due to a damaged mitral valve

Z2. drawing blood from a vein via a small incision

A3. sudden drop in the supply of blood to an area of the heart muscle, usually due to a blockage in a coronary artery

B3. buildup of solid material, such as a fatty deposit, on the lining of an artery

C3. surgical replacement of a coronary valve

D3. viewing of the heart by magnetic resonance imaging

E3. heart disease (usually a type of malformation) that exists at birth

F3. abnormal narrowing of the opening of the tricuspid valve

G3. process of passing a thin catheter through an artery or vein to the heart to take blood samples, inject a contrast medium, or measure various pressures

H3. percentage of the volume of the contents of the left ventricle ejected

___ 69. peripheral vascular disease

___ 70. lumen

___ 71. petechiae

___ 72. mitral valve

___ 73. valve replacement

___ 74. anastomosis

___ 75. thrombectomy

___ 76. intracardiac tumor

___ 77. aortography

___ 78. myocardial infarction

___ 79. electrocardiography

___ 80. echocardiography

___ 81. venule

___ 82. endothelium

___ 83. cholesterol

___ 84. cyanosis

___ 85. arteriosclerosis

___ 86. cardiac tamponade

___ 87. high blood pressure

___ 88. heart

___ 89. embolus

___ 90. venography

___ 91. cardiac enzyme tests/studies

___ 92. fibrillation

___ 93. embolectomy

___ 94. right atrium

___ 95. tetralogy of fallot

___ 96. carotid artery

___ 97. serum enzyme tests

___ 98. phlebotomy

___ 99. artery

___ 100. hypertensive heart disease

___ 101. hypotension

___ 102. murmur

___ 103. cardiac cycle

___ 104. aorta

___ 105. atherectomy

___ 106. heart transplant

with each contraction

I3. death of tissue or an organ part due to irreversible damage; usually a result of oxygen deprivation

J3. *see bypass

K3. sound or murmur, especially an abnormal heart sound heard on auscultation, especially of the carotid artery

L3. procedure that uses a balloon catheter to open narrowed orifices in cardiac valves

M3. viewing of a vein by x-ray after injection of a contrast medium

N3. chest pain, usually caused by a lowered oxygen or blood supply to the heart

O3. atrioventricular valve on the right side of the heart

P3. any of various blood vessels carrying deoxygenated blood toward the heart, except the pulmonary vein

Q3. narrowing of the aorta

R3. minute hemorrhages in the skin

S3. opening of a blocked blood vessel, as by balloon dilation

T3. surgical removal of a thrombus

U3. a thick-walled blood vessel that, in systemic circulation, carries oxygenated blood away from the heart

V3. waste material transported in the venous blood

W3. a tiny artery connecting to a capillary

X3. frictional sound heard between heartbeats, usually indication a pericardial murmur

Y3. large vein that transports blood collected from the upper part of the body to the heart

Z3. surgical reconstruction of a cardiac valve

A4. viewing of the interior o f a blood vessel using a fiberoptic catheter inserted or threaded into the vessel

B4. the closing of a blood vessel

C4. set of four congenital heart abnormalities appearing together that cause deoxygenated blood to enter the systemic circulation: ventricular septal defect, pulmonary stenosis, incorrect position of the aorta, and rich ventricular hypertrophy

D4. channel inside an artery through which blood flows

E4. production of images based on the echoes of sound waves against structures

F4. formation of a thrombus (clot) in a deep vein, such as a femoral vein

G4. either of the two lower chambers of the heart

H4. portable device that provides a 24-hour electrocardiogram

I4. the smallest blood vessel that forms the exchange point between the arterial and venous vessels

J4. compression or narrowing caused by contraction, as of a vessel

K4. one of four veins that bring oxygenated blood from the lungs to the

___ 107. plaque

___ 108. congenital heart disease

___ 109. pulse

___ 110. angioscopy

___ 111. pacemaker

___ 112. popliteal artery

___ 113. coarctation of the aorta

___ 114. multiple-gated acquisition (MUGA) angiography

___ 115. varicose vein

___ 116. thrombotic occlusion

___ 117. pericarditis

___ 118. lipid profile

___ 119. left atrium

___ 120. triglyceride

___ 121. ventricle

___ 122. inferior vena cava

___ 123. arteriole

___ 124. aortic stenosis

___ 125. valve

___ 126. endocardium

___ 127. percutaneous trans luminal coronary angioplasty

___ 128. vein

___ 129. bicuspid valve

___ 130. perfusion deficit

___ 131. ischemia

___ 132. angina

___ 133. cardiac MRI

___ 134. occlusion

___ 135. premature ventricular contractions (PVCs)

___ 136. bradycardia

___ 137. cardiopulmonary bypass

left atrium

L4. surgical removal of hemorrhoids

M4. any tissue or organ implanted to replace or mend damaged areas

N4. *see bicuspid valve

O4. compression of the heart caused by fluid accumulation in the pericardial sac

P4. any of the tubular passageways in the cardiovascular system through which blood travels

Q4. radioactive scan showing heart function

R4. region of the right atrium containing specialized tissue that sends electrical impulses to the heart muscle, causing it to contract

S4. inflammation of the myocardium

T4. narrowing of the pulmonary artery, preventing the lungs from receiving enough blood from the heart to oxygenate

U4. mass of foreign material blocking a vessel

V4. inflammation of a vein

W4. any of various factors considered to increase the probability that a disease will occur; for example, high blood pressure and smoking are considered risk factors for heart disease

X4. viewing of a specific artery by x-ray after injection of a contrast medium

Y4. incision into a cardiac valve to remove an obstruction

Z4. *see atrioventricular block

A5. essential fluid made up of plasma & other elements that circulates throughout the body; delivers nutrients to and removes waste from the body's cells

B5. varicose condition of veins in the anal region

C5. surgical procedure that creates a bypass from the right atrium to the main pulmonary artery; fontal's procedure

D5. inflammation of a heart valve

E5. an irregular, usually rapid, heartbeat caused by overstimulation of the AV node

F5. upper right chamber of the heart

G5. *see hypotension

H5. lower right chamber of the heart

I5. contracting state of the myocardial tissue in the heart's conduction system

J5. angina pectoris

K5. valve between the aorta and the left ventricle

L5. viewing of a vein by x-ray after injection of a contrast medium

M5. spasm in the arteries of the fingers causing numbness or pain

N5. a condition at birth in which the ductus arteriousus, a small duct between the aorta and the pulmonary artery, remains abnormally open

_____ 138. rub

_____ 139. patent ductus arteriosus

_____ 140. angioplasty

_____ 141. vena cava (p. venae cavae)

_____ 142. bacterial endocarditis

_____ 143. secondary hypertension

_____ 144. epicardium

_____ 145. ductus venosus

_____ 146. flutter

_____ 147. stenosis

_____ 148. endovascular surgery

_____ 149. positron emission tomography (PET) scan

_____ 150. mitral insufficiency / reflux

_____ 151. foramen ovale

_____ 152. atrium (p. atria)

_____ 153. gallop

_____ 154. coronary bypass surgery

_____ 155. sinus rhythm

_____ 156. left ventricle

_____ 157. pulmonary valve

_____ 158. valvotomy

_____ 159. coronary artery

_____ 160. palpitations

_____ 161. pulmonary artery

_____ 162. septum (p. septa)

_____ 163. thrombus

_____ 164. polarization

_____ 165. conduction system

_____ 166. valvulitis

_____ 167. super vena cava

_____ 168. atrioventricular (AV) node

_____ 169. graft

O5. one of the two valves that prevent the back flow of blood flowing out of the heart into the aorta and the pulmonary artery

P5. structure in the fetal circulatory system through which blood flows to bypass the fetal liver

Q5. inflammation of the pericardium

R5. condition that reduces the flow of blood and nutrients through the arteries of the heart

S5. artery that transports oxygenated blood to the head and neck

T5. uncomfortable pulsations of the heart felt as a thumping in the chest

U5. outermost layer of heart tissue

V5. structure in the fetal circulatory system through which blood flows to bypass the fetus's nonfunctioning lungs

W5. fatty substance; lipid

X5. blood vessel that supplies oxygen-rich blood to the heart

Y5. muscular layer of heart tissue between the epicardium and the endocardium

Z5. abnormal accumulation of fluid in the lungs

A6. heart rate greater than 100 beats per minute

B6. localized blood insufficiency caused by an obstruction

C6. term for the sinoatrial (SA) node; also, an artificial device that regulates heart rhythm

D6. procedure used during surgery to divert blood flow to and from the heart through a heart- lung machine and back into circulation

E6. Relating to or affecting the heart and blood vessels.

F6. lack of flow through a blood vessel, usually caused by an occlusion

G6. inflammation of an artery or arteries

H6. either of the two upper chambers of the heart

I6. backward flow of blood into the left atrium due to protrusion of one or both mitral cusps into the left atrium during contractions

J6. process of viewing the heart muscle at work by scanning the heart of a patient into whom a radioactive substance has been injected

K6. attacks of limping, particularly in the legs, due to ischemia of the muscles

L6. fatty substance present in animal fats; cholesterol circulates int the bloodstream, sometimes causing arterial plaque to form

M6. surgical removal of an embolus

N6. ballooning of the artery wall caused by weakness in the wall

O6. vascular disease in the lower extremities, usually due to the blockages in the arteries of the groin or legs

P6. narrowing caused by a thrombus

Q6. triple sound of a heartbeat, usually indicative of serious heart disease

R6. measure of the force of blood surging against the walls of the arteries

_____ 170. infarction

_____ 171. right ventricle

_____ 172. mitral valve prolapse

_____ 173. atrial fibrillation

_____ 174. rheumatic heart disease

_____ 175. valvuloplasty

_____ 176. stress test

_____ 177. cardiac scan

_____ 178. bypass

_____ 179. blood

_____ 180. phlebography

_____ 181. atheroma

_____ 182. balloon catheter dilation

_____ 183. auscultation

_____ 184. digital subtraction angiography

_____ 185. infarct

_____ 186. blood vessel

_____ 187. myocarditis

_____ 188. thrombosis

_____ 189. stent

_____ 190. aortic valve

_____ 191. thrombophlebitis

_____ 192. essential hypertension

_____ 193. claudication

_____ 194. bruit

_____ 195. low blood pressure

_____ 196. pericardium

S6. narrowing, particularly of blood vessels or of the cardiac valves

T6. test that measures heart rate, blood pressure, and other body functions while the patient is exercising on a treadmill

U6. small puncture into a vein, usually to draw blood or inject a solution

V6. bacterial inflammation of the inner lining of the heart

W6. contraction phase of the heartbeat

X6. congenital abnormality consisting of an opening in the septum between the atria or ventricles

Y6. soft heart humming sound heard between normal beats

Z6. heart block; partial or complete blockage of the electrical impulses from the atrioventricular node to the ventricles

A7. a fatty deposit (plaque) in the wall of an artery

B7. atrial contractions that occur before the normal impulse; can be the cause of palpitations

C7. lower left heart chamber

D7. heart rate of fewer then 60 beats per minute

E7. device for measuring blood pressure

F7. bundle of fivers in the inter ventricular septum that transfers charges in the heart's conduction system; also called bundle of His

G7. stationary blood clot in the cardiovascular system, usually formed from matter found in the blood

H7. a tumor within one of the heart chambers

I7. muscular organ that receives blood from the veins and sends it into the arteries

J7. laboratory tests performed to detect enzymes present during or after a myocardial infarction; cardiac enzyme studies

K7. any of a group of veins that transport deoxygenated blood from the legs

L7. backward flow or leakage of blood through a faulty aortic valve

M7. resting state of the myocardial tissue in the conduction system of the heart

N7. repeated contraction and relaxation of the heart as it circulates blood within itself and pumps it out to the rest of the body or the lungs

O7. use of sound waves to produce images showing the structure and motion of the heart

P7. part of the heart containing specialized tissue that sends electrical charges through heart fibers, causing the heart to contract and relax at regular intervals

Q7. any of various procedures performed during cardiac catheterization, such as angioscopy and atherectomy

R7. protective covering of the heart

S7. viewing of the heart's major blood vessels by x-ray after injection of a contrast medium

T7. hardening of the arteries

U7. regular but very rapid heartbeat

V7. rhythmic expansion and contraction of a blood vessel, usually an artery

W7. hypertension having a known cause, such as kidney disease

X7. insertion of a balloon catheter into a blood vessel to open the passage so blood can flow freely

Y7. *see angioplasty

Z7. any of various structures that slow or prevent fluid from flowing backward or forward

A8. abnormal heart rhythm

B8. a structure (usually a vein graft) that creates a new passage for blood flow from one artery to another artery or part of an artery; used to create a detour around blockages in the arteries

C8. membranous lining of the chambers and valves of the heart; the innermost layer of heart tissue

D8. a tiny vein connecting to a capillary

E8. partition between the left and right chambers of the heart

F8. ventricular contractions that occur before the normal impulse; can be the cause of palpitations

G8. recharging state; transition from contraction to resting that occurs in the conduction system of the heart

H8. abnormal narrowing of the aorta

I8. *see balloon catheter dilation

J8. surgical incision into an artery, especially to remove a clot

K8. specialized part of the interatrial septum that sends a charge to the bundle of His

L8. *see superior vena cava & inferior vena cava

M8. opening in the septum of the fetal heart that closes at birth

N8. use of the electrocardiograph in diagnosis

Terminology #6 Quiz

Circle the letter of the Definition that corresponds to the displayed Term.

1. septal defect

    A. waste material transported in the venous blood

    B. stationary blood clot in the cardiovascular system, usually formed from matter found in the blood

    C. ultrasound test of blood flow in certain blood vessels

    D. congenital abnormality consisting of an opening in the septum between the atria or ventricles

2. ventriculogram

    A. an artery that supplies blood to the thigh

    B. backward flow of blood due to a damaged mitral valve

    C. Relating to or affecting the heart and blood vessels.

    D. x-ray of a ventricle taken after injection of a contrast medium

3. asystole

    A. blood vessel that supplies oxygen-rich blood to the heart

    B. congenital abnormality consisting of an opening in the septum between the atria or ventricles

    C. compression or narrowing caused by contraction, as of a vessel

    D. cardiac arrest

4. arteritis

    A. heart valve and/or muscle damage caused by an untreated streptococcal infection

    B. chest pain, usually caused by a lowered oxygen or blood supply to the heart

    C. inflammation of an artery or arteries

    D. limping caused by inadequate blood supply during activity; usually subsides during rest

5. pulmonary valve

    A. resting state of the myocardial tissue in the conduction system of the heart

    B. valve that controls the blood flow between the right ventricle and the pulmonary arteries

    C. hypertension having a known cause, such as kidney disease

    D. channel inside an artery through which blood flows

6. phlebotomy

    A. outermost layer of heart tissue

    B. essential fluid made up of plasma & other elements that circulates throughout the body; delivers nutrients to and removes waste from the body's cells

    C. drawing blood from a vein via a small incision

    D. limping caused by inadequate blood supply during activity; usually subsides during rest

7. sinoatrial (SA) node

A. test that measures heart rate, blood pressure, and other body functions while the patient is exercising on a treadmill

B. surgical removal of an atheroma

C. region of the right atrium containing specialized tissue that sends electrical impulses to the heart muscle, causing it to contract

D. surgical removal of an embolus

8. triglyceride

A. a tiny vein connecting to a capillary

B. surgical removal of hemorrhoids

C. either of the two lower chambers of the heart

D. fatty substance; lipid

9. atrioventricular valve

A. surgical incision into an artery, especially to remove a clot

B. one of two valves that control blood flow between the atria and ventricles

C. sound or murmur, especially an abnormal heart sound heard on auscultation, especially of the carotid artery

D. any of various factors considered to increase the probability that a disease will occur; for example, high blood pressure and smoking are considered risk factors for heart disease

10. arteriosclerosis

A. partition between the left and right chambers of the heart

B. drawing blood from a vein via a small incision

C. hardening of the arteries

D. radioactive scan showing heart function

Circle the letter of the Term that corresponds to the displayed Definition.

11. partition between the left and right chambers of the heart

A. septum (p. septa)

B. heart transplant

C. epicardium

D. vena cava (p. venae cavae)

12. surgically implanted devices used to hold something (as a blood vessel) open

A. aortic valve

B. stent

C. pulmonary artery

D. angiography

13. viewing of the heart's major blood vessels by x-ray after injection of a contrast medium

A. blood pressure

B. aortography

C. bicuspid valve

D. angiography

14. muscular organ that receives blood from the veins and sends it into the arteries

    A. heart

    B. bundle of His

    C. capillary

    D. percutaneous trans luminal coronary angioplasty

15. blood tests for determining levels of enzymes during a myocardial infarction; serum enzyme tests

    A. intracardiac tumor

    B. cholesterol

    C. cardiac enzyme tests/studies

    D. angiocardiography

16. stent placed within a blood vessel to allow blood to flow freely

    A. intravascular stent

    B. intermittent claudication

    C. carotid artery

    D. serum enzyme tests

17. small puncture into a vein, usually to draw blood or inject a solution

    A. echocardiography

    B. venipuncture

    C. mitral valve

    D. lipid profile

18. sudden drop in the supply of arterial or venous blood, often due to an embolus or thrombus

    A. infarction

    B. arteriosclerosis

    C. diastole

    D. arrhythmia

19. *see bicuspid valve

    A. coronary angioplasty

    B. ventriculogram

    C. doppler ultrasound

    D. mitral valve

20. an artery that supplies blood to the thigh

    A. coronary artery disease

    B. phlebotomy

C. atrium (p. atria)

D. femoral artery

EXTRA CREDIT: Give the Term that corresponds to the displayed Definition.

21. viewing of a vein by x-ray after injection of a contrast medium

Terminology #6 Test

Enter the letter for the matching Definition

1. ☐ embolus
2. ☐ fontan's operation
3. ☐ gallop
4. ☐ deep vein thrombosis
5. ☐ endovascular surgery
6. ☐ systole
7. ☐ varicose vein
8. ☐ venule
9. ☐ coarctation of the aorta
10. ☐ ventriculogram
11. ☐ atrium (p. atria)
12. ☐ angioplasty
13. ☐ valve
14. ☐ dysrhythmia
15. ☐ carotid artery
16. ☐ saphenous vein
17. ☐ cardiomyopathy
18. ☐ electrocardiography
19. ☐ aortography
20. ☐ peripheral vascular disease

A. abnormal narrowing of the aorta

B. dilated, enlarged, or twisted vein, usually on the leg

C. triple sound of a heartbeat, usually indicative of serious heart disease

D. surgical procedure that creates a bypass from the right atrium to the main pulmonary artery; fontal's procedure

E. artery that transports oxygenated blood to the head and neck

F. x-ray of a ventricle taken after injection of a contrast medium

G. any of various procedures performed during cardiac catheterization, such as angioscopy and atherectomy

H. contraction phase of the heartbeat

I. vascular disease in the lower extremities, usually due to the blockages in the arteries of the groin or legs

J. either of the two upper chambers of the heart

K. any of a group of veins that transport deoxygenated blood from the legs

L. viewing of the aorta by x-ray after injection of a contrast medium

M. any of various structures that slow or prevent fluid from flowing backward or forward

N. opening of a blocked blood vessel, as by balloon dilation

O. use of the electrocardiograph in diagnosis

P. abnormal heart rhythm

Q. a tiny vein connecting to a capillary

R. formation of a thrombus (clot) in a deep vein, such as a femoral vein

S. disease of the heart muscle

T. mass of foreign material blocking a vessel

Give the Definition that corresponds to the displayed Term.

21. triglyceride

Give the Term that corresponds to the displayed Definition.

22. muscular organ that receives blood from the veins and sends it into the arteries

23. viewing of the heart and its major blood vessels by x-ray after injection of a contrast medium

24. a fatty deposit (plaque) in the wall of an artery

25. hardening of the arteries

26. narrowing of the pulmonary artery, preventing the lungs from receiving enough blood from the heart to oxygenate

27. uncomfortable pulsations of the heart felt as a thumping in the chest

28. viewing of the interior o f a blood vessel using a fiberoptic catheter inserted or threaded into the vessel

29. localized blood insufficiency caused by an obstruction

30. procedure that uses a balloon catheter to open narrowed orifices in cardiac valves

B	I	N	G	O
fontan's operation	ductus venosus	cardiac tamponade	cholesterol	carbon dioxide
peripheral vascular disease	coronary bypass surgery	intravascular stent	depolarization	occlusion
angina pectoris	septal defect	FREE	intracardiac tumor	fibrillation
secondary hypertension	mitral stenosis	mitral valve prolapse	venipuncture	petechiae
atrioventricular valve	constriction	hypertensive heart disease	deep vein thrombosis	embolus

B	I	N	G	O
sinus rhythm	semilunar valve	foramen ovale	inferior vena cava	vegetation
right ventricle	venipuncture	digital subtraction angiography	constriction	stent
pulmonary artery	atrioventricular valve	FREE	fontan's operation	atherosclerosis
mitral insufficiency / reflux	phlebitis	premature atrial contractions (PACs)	electrocardiography	plaque
hypertension	polarization	high blood pressure	arrhythmia	blood vessel

B	I	N	G	O
left atrium	heart transplant	pacemaker	pericardium	polarization
patent ductus arteriosus	myocarditis	positron emission tomography (PET) scan	atrioventricular block	percutaneous trans luminal coronary angioplasty
valve replacement	gallop	FREE	venography	hemorrhoidectomy
embolectomy	rub	septum (p. septa)	plaque	femoral artery
blood	phlebography	valve	pulmonary vein	sinoatrial (SA) node

BINGO

B	I	N	G	O
raynaud's phenomenon	stenosis	triglyceride	bradycardia	artery
gallop	rheumatic heart disease	right ventricle	cardiac MRI	mitral valve
pulmonary vein	electrocardiography	FREE	aortic valve	essential hypertension
blood vessel	conduction system	flutter	sphygmomanometer	holter monitor
cholesterol	endothelium	valve replacement	fibrillation	hemorrhoid

B	I	N	G	O
arteriole	endocardium	pericarditits	rub	depolarization
phlebography	mitral insufficiency / reflux	aortic regurgitation	angioscopy	risk factor
high blood pressure	phlebitis	FREE	foramen ovale	raynaud's phenomenon
polarization	congenital heart disease	premature atrial contractions (PACs)	bundle of His	tricuspid stenosis
angina pectoris	pulmonary vein	vena cava (p. venae cavae)	flutter	coronary bypass surgery

B	I	N	G	O
endarterectomy	hypertension	angina pectoris	mitral valve prolapse	flutter
hemorrhoidectomy	mitral insufficiency / reflux	bruit	hemorrhoid	carotid artery
bradycardia	tricuspid stenosis	FREE	pulmonary artery	intracardiac tumor
heart	angiocardiography	aortic regurgitation	cardiopulmonary bypass	aorta
hypertensive heart disease	cardiomyopathy	bicuspid valve	coronary artery	angioplasty

B	I	N	G	O
cardiac tamponade	left atrium	arteriography	atheroma	angiocardiography
premature atrial contractions (PACs)	myocardium	stenosis	mitral stenosis	cholesterol
hypertensive heart disease	deep vein thrombosis	FREE	serum enzyme tests	atherectomy
phlebotomy	bundle of His	sinoatrial (SA) node	tricuspid stenosis	thrombotic occlusion
percutaneous trans luminal coronary angioplasty	mitral valve prolapse	myocardial infarction	valve replacement	ductus arteriousus

B I N G O

septal defect	secondary hypertension	stenosis	cardiopulmonary bypass	rub
embolus	dysrhythmia	petechiae	myocardium	pulmonary artery
bradycardia	phlebotomy	FREE	bruit	arteriole
atherectomy	ischemia	rheumatic heart disease	raynaud's phenomenon	angioplasty
myocardial infarction	atrioventricular bundle	saphenous vein	venipuncture	hypertensive heart disease

B	I	N	G	O
hemorrhoidectomy	positron emission tomography (PET) scan	pulmonary valve	myocardial infarction	artery
perfusion deficit	myocardium	pericarditits	cardiac cycle	fibrillation
necrosis	angina	FREE	constriction	embolectomy
cardiopulmonary bypass	valve replacement	peripheral vascular disease	holter monitor	right ventricle
plaque	septum (p. septa)	vena cava (p. venae cavae)	aortic stenosis	vein

B	I	N	G	O
embolectomy	pulmonary vein	aorta	angiography	risk factor
angioscopy	arteriography	aortic regurgitation	vena cava (p. venae cavae)	petechiae
cardiac scan	epicardium	FREE	thrombotic occlusion	atrial fibrillation
high blood pressure	thrombectomy	left ventricle	repolarization	cardiac catheterization
aortic stenosis	aortography	bacterial endocarditis	doppler ultrasound	palpitations

B	I	N	G	O
stent	capillary	myocarditis	murmur	hypotension
premature ventricular contractions (PVCs)	cardiac enzyme tests/studies	vegetation	diastole	hemorrhoid
left ventricle	repolarization	FREE	premature atrial contractions (PACs)	pericarditits
arteritis	asystole	atrioventricular bundle	artery	angiography
venule	balloon catheter dilation	fibrillation	systole	coarctation of the aorta

B	I	N	G	O
cardiac tamponade	bacterial endocarditis	high blood pressure	endovascular surgery	blood
endocarditis	electrocardiography	vegetation	bundle of His	deep vein thrombosis
cholesterol	right ventricle	FREE	polarization	atherectomy
endarterectomy	heart block	echocardiography	petechiae	angiography
cyanosis	hypertensive heart disease	foramen ovale	raynaud's phenomenon	auscultation

B	I	N	G	O
echocardiography	pericardium	perfusion deficit	rheumatic heart disease	ischemia
patent ductus arteriosus	percutaneous trans luminal coronary angioplasty	stent	cardiac cycle	atheroma
graft	necrosis	FREE	diastole	venule
femoral artery	heart	valvotomy	aneurysm	atrium (p. atria)
endarterectomy	venipuncture	pulse	septal defect	left atrium

B	I	N	G	O
stent	pulmonary valve	tachycardia	angina	tricuspid stenosis
valvuloplasty	conduction system	right ventricle	angioscopy	murmur
ischemia	valve replacement	FREE	congenital heart disease	cardiac cycle
polarization	fibrillation	pulmonary edema	atrioventricular valve	phlebotomy
premature ventricular contractions (PVCs)	carbon dioxide	necrosis	ejection fraction	heart block

B	I	N	G	O
pulmonary vein	fontan's operation	cardiac enzyme tests/studies	ductus arteriousus	vein
serum enzyme tests	rheumatic heart disease	sphygmomanometer	infarction	peripheral vascular disease
semilunar valve	patent ductus arteriosus	FREE	arteriole	hemorrhoidectomy
aortic regurgitation	pulmonary valve	coronary bypass surgery	arteriosclerosis	coarctation of the aorta
blood	balloon valvuloplasty	myocarditis	necrosis	blood pressure

B	I	N	G	O
valve	ejection fraction	aortic stenosis	cardiomyopathy	capillary
endocardium	venography	pulmonary artery stenosis	pacemaker	arteriotomy
lumen	mitral valve prolapse	FREE	balloon valvuloplasty	angiography
sphygmomanometer	cyanosis	multiple-gated acquisition (MUGA) angiography	serum enzyme tests	stent
popliteal artery	cholesterol	cardiopulmonary bypass	percutaneous trans luminal coronary angioplasty	sinoatrial (SA) node

B	I	N	G	O
serum enzyme tests	palpitations	cardiac catheterization	popliteal artery	arteriosclerosis
rheumatic heart disease	hypertensive heart disease	digital subtraction angiography	lumen	repolarization
perfusion deficit	sonography	FREE	aortic regurgitation	tetralogy of fallot
coarctation of the aorta	aneurysm	arteriography	angina	vein
cardiopulmonary bypass	angiocardiography	atrioventricular valve	bruit	necrosis

B	I	N	G	O
secondary hypertension	serum enzyme tests	carbon dioxide	cyanosis	ventriculogram
epicardium	foramen ovale	endothelium	inferior vena cava	cardiac catheterization
angina	multiple-gated acquisition (MUGA) angiography	FREE	lumen	cardiovascular
depolarization	blood	murmur	holter monitor	bypass
tetralogy of fallot	arteriole	aorta	conduction system	rheumatic heart disease

B	I	N	G	O
conduction system	fibrillation	arteritis	depolarization	doppler ultrasound
cardiac enzyme tests/studies	heart	percutaneous trans luminal coronary angioplasty	venography	pulmonary artery
coronary artery	aortic regurgitation	FREE	ischemia	bruit
atrial fibrillation	atrium (p. atria)	phlebotomy	heart transplant	vegetation
valve replacement	arteriography	endothelium	semilunar valve	phlebography

B	I	N	G	O
tetralogy of fallot	intravascular stent	stress test	aortic stenosis	diastole
pulmonary artery stenosis	plaque	atheroma	cardiomyopathy	right ventricle
carbon dioxide	cardiac arrest	FREE	serum enzyme tests	tachycardia
flutter	pericardium	holter monitor	foramen ovale	pulmonary artery
arteriosclerosis	femoral artery	secondary hypertension	lipid profile	heart transplant

B	I	N	G	O	
B	I	N	G	O	largest artery of the body; vessel through which oxygenated blood exits the heart
B	I	N	G	O	valve between the aorta and the left ventricle
B	I	N	G	O	a tiny artery connecting to a capillary
B	I	N	G	O	a thick-walled blood vessel that, in systemic circulation, carries oxygenated blood away from the heart
B	I	N	G	O	bundle of fivers in the inter ventricular septum that transfers charges in the heart's conduction system; also called bundle of His
B	I	N	G	O	specialized part of the interatrial septum that sends a charge to the bundle of His
B	I	N	G	O	one of two valves that control blood flow between the atria and ventricles
B	I	N	G	O	either of the two upper chambers of the heart
B	I	N	G	O	atrioventricular valve on the left side of the heart
B	I	N	G	O	essential fluid made up of plasma & other elements that circulates throughout the body; delivers nutrients to and removes waste from the body's cells
B	I	N	G	O	measure of the force of blood surging against the walls of the arteries
B	I	N	G	O	any of the tubular passageways in the cardiovascular system through which blood travels
B	I	N	G	O	*see atrioventricular bundle
B	I	N	G	O	the smallest blood vessel that forms the exchange point between the arterial and venous vessels
B	I	N	G	O	waste material transported in the venous blood
B	I	N	G	O	repeated contraction and relaxation of the heart as it circulates blood within itself and pumps it out to the rest of the body or the lungs
B	I	N	G	O	Relating to or affecting the heart and blood vessels.
B	I	N	G	O	artery that transports oxygenated blood to the head and neck
B	I	N	G	O	part of the heart containing specialized tissue that sends electrical charges through heart fibers, causing the heart to contract and relax at regular intervals
B	I	N	G	O	blood vessel that supplies oxygen-rich blood to the heart
B	I	N	G	O	contracting state of the myocardial tissue in the heart's conduction system
B	I	N	G	O	relaxation phase of a heartbeat
B	I	N	G	O	structure in the fetal circulatory system through which blood flows to bypass the fetus's nonfunctioning lungs
B	I	N	G	O	structure in the fetal circulatory system through which blood flows to bypass the fetal liver
B	I	N	G	O	membranous lining of the chambers and valves of the heart; the innermost layer of heart tissue
B	I	N	G	O	lining of the arteries that secretes substances into the blood
B	I	N	G	O	outermost layer of heart tissue
B	I	N	G	O	an artery that supplies blood to the thigh
B	I	N	G	O	opening in the septum of the fetal heart that closes at birth
B	I	N	G	O	muscular organ that receives blood from the veins and sends it into the arteries
B	I	N	G	O	large vein that draws blood from the lower part of the body to the right atrium
B	I	N	G	O	upper left heart chamber
B	I	N	G	O	lower left heart chamber
B	I	N	G	O	channel inside an artery through which blood flows
B	I	N	G	O	*see bicuspid valve
B	I	N	G	O	muscular layer of heart tissue between the epicardium and the endocardium
B	I	N	G	O	term for the sinoatrial (SA) node; also, an artificial device that regulates heart rhythm
B	I	N	G	O	protective covering of the heart
B	I	N	G	O	resting state of the myocardial tissue in the conduction system of the heart
B	I	N	G	O	an artery that supplies blood to the cells of the area behind the knee

B	I	N	G	O	
B	I	N	G	O	one of two arteries that carry blood that is low in oxygen from the heart to the lungs
B	I	N	G	O	valve that controls the blood flow between the right ventricle and the pulmonary arteries
B	I	N	G	O	one of four veins that bring oxygenated blood from the lungs to the left atrium
B	I	N	G	O	rhythmic expansion and contraction of a blood vessel, usually an artery
B	I	N	G	O	recharging state; transition from contraction to resting that occurs in the conduction system of the heart
B	I	N	G	O	upper right chamber of the heart
B	I	N	G	O	lower right chamber of the heart
B	I	N	G	O	any of a group of veins that transport deoxygenated blood from the legs
B	I	N	G	O	one of the two valves that prevent the back flow of blood flowing out of the heart into the aorta and the pulmonary artery
B	I	N	G	O	partition between the left and right chambers of the heart
B	I	N	G	O	region of the right atrium containing specialized tissue that sends electrical impulses to the heart muscle, causing it to contract
B	I	N	G	O	normal heart rhythm
B	I	N	G	O	large vein that transports blood collected from the upper part of the body to the heart
B	I	N	G	O	contraction phase of the heartbeat
B	I	N	G	O	atrioventricular valve on the right side of the heart
B	I	N	G	O	any of various structures that slow or prevent fluid from flowing backward or forward
B	I	N	G	O	any of various blood vessels carrying deoxygenated blood toward the heart, except the pulmonary vein
B	I	N	G	O	*see superior vena cava & inferior vena cava
B	I	N	G	O	either of the two lower chambers of the heart
B	I	N	G	O	a tiny vein connecting to a capillary
B	I	N	G	O	viewing of the heart and its major blood vessels by x-ray after injection of a contrast medium
B	I	N	G	O	viewing of the heart's major blood vessels by x-ray after injection of a contrast medium
B	I	N	G	O	viewing of the aorta by x-ray after injection of a contrast medium
B	I	N	G	O	viewing of a specific artery by x-ray after injection of a contrast medium
B	I	N	G	O	process of listening to body sounds via a stethoscope
B	I	N	G	O	process of passing a thin catheter through an artery or vein to the heart to take blood samples, inject a contrast medium, or measure various pressures
B	I	N	G	O	blood tests for determining levels of enzymes during a myocardial infarction; serum enzyme tests
B	I	N	G	O	viewing of the heart by magnetic resonance imaging
B	I	N	G	O	process of viewing the heart muscle at work by scanning the heart of a patient into whom a radioactive substance has been injected
B	I	N	G	O	fatty substance present in animal fats; cholesterol circulates int the bloodstream, sometimes causing arterial plaque to form
B	I	N	G	O	use of two angiograms done with different dyes to provide a comparison between the results
B	I	N	G	O	ultrasound test of blood flow in certain blood vessels
B	I	N	G	O	use of sound waves to produce images showing the structure and motion of the heart
B	I	N	G	O	percentage of the volume of the contents of the left ventricle ejected with each contraction
B	I	N	G	O	use of the electrocardiograph in diagnosis
B	I	N	G	O	portable device that provides a 24-hour electrocardiogram
B	I	N	G	O	laboratory test that provides the levels of lipids, triglycerides, and other substances in the blood
B	I	N	G	O	radioactive scan showing heart function
B	I	N	G	O	viewing of a vein by x-ray after injection of a contrast medium

B	I	N	G	O	
B	I	N	G	O	type of nuclear image that measures movement of areas of the heart
B	I	N	G	O	laboratory tests performed to detect enzymes present during or after a myocardial infarction; cardiac enzyme studies
B	I	N	G	O	production of images based on the echoes of sound waves against structures
B	I	N	G	O	device for measuring blood pressure
B	I	N	G	O	test that measures heart rate, blood pressure, and other body functions while the patient is exercising on a treadmill
B	I	N	G	O	fatty substance; lipid
B	I	N	G	O	viewing of a vein by x-ray after injection of a contrast medium
B	I	N	G	O	x-ray of a ventricle taken after injection of a contrast medium
B	I	N	G	O	ballooning of the artery wall caused by weakness in the wall
B	I	N	G	O	angina pectoris
B	I	N	G	O	chest pain, usually caused by a lowered oxygen or blood supply to the heart
B	I	N	G	O	backward flow or leakage of blood through a faulty aortic valve
B	I	N	G	O	narrowing of the aorta
B	I	N	G	O	irregularity in the rhythm of the heartbeat
B	I	N	G	O	hardening of the arteries
B	I	N	G	O	inflammation of an artery or arteries
B	I	N	G	O	cardiac arrest
B	I	N	G	O	a fatty deposit (plaque) in the wall of an artery
B	I	N	G	O	hardening of the arteries caused by the buildup of atheromas
B	I	N	G	O	an irregular, usually rapid, heartbeat caused by overstimulation of the AV node
B	I	N	G	O	heart block; partial or complete blockage of the electrical impulses from the atrioventricular node to the ventricles
B	I	N	G	O	bacterial inflammation of the inner lining of the heart
B	I	N	G	O	heart rate of fewer then 60 beats per minute
B	I	N	G	O	sound or murmur, especially an abnormal heart sound heard on auscultation, especially of the carotid artery
B	I	N	G	O	sudden stopping of the heart; also called asystole
B	I	N	G	O	compression of the heart caused by fluid accumulation in the pericardial sac
B	I	N	G	O	disease of the heart muscle
B	I	N	G	O	limping caused by inadequate blood supply during activity; usually subsides during rest
B	I	N	G	O	abnormal narrowing of the aorta
B	I	N	G	O	heart disease (usually a type of malformation) that exists at birth
B	I	N	G	O	compression or narrowing caused by contraction, as of a vessel
B	I	N	G	O	condition that reduces the flow of blood and nutrients through the arteries of the heart
B	I	N	G	O	bluish or purplish coloration, as of the skin, caused by inadequate oxygenation of the blood
B	I	N	G	O	formation of a thrombus (clot) in a deep vein, such as a femoral vein
B	I	N	G	O	abnormal heart rhythm
B	I	N	G	O	mass of foreign material blocking a vessel
B	I	N	G	O	inflammation of the endocardium, especially an inflammation caused by a bacterial or fungal agent
B	I	N	G	O	high blood pressure without any known cause
B	I	N	G	O	random, chaotic, irregular heart rhythm
B	I	N	G	O	regular but very rapid heartbeat
B	I	N	G	O	triple sound of a heartbeat, usually indicative of serious heart disease
B	I	N	G	O	*see atrioventricular block

B	I	N	G	O	
B	I	N	G	O	varicose condition of veins in the anal region
B	I	N	G	O	*see hypertension
B	I	N	G	O	chronic condition with blood pressure greater than 140/90
B	I	N	G	O	heart disease caused, or worsened, by high blood pressure
B	I	N	G	O	chronic condition with blood pressure below normal
B	I	N	G	O	area of necrosis caused by a sudden drop in the supply of arterial or venous blood
B	I	N	G	O	sudden drop in the supply of arterial or venous blood, often due to an embolus or thrombus
B	I	N	G	O	attacks of limping, particularly in the legs, due to ischemia of the muscles
B	I	N	G	O	a tumor within one of the heart chambers
B	I	N	G	O	localized blood insufficiency caused by an obstruction
B	I	N	G	O	*see hypotension
B	I	N	G	O	backward flow of blood due to a damaged mitral valve
B	I	N	G	O	abnormal narrowing at the opening of the mitral valve
B	I	N	G	O	backward flow of blood into the left atrium due to protrusion of one or both mitral cusps into the left atrium during contractions
B	I	N	G	O	soft heart humming sound heard between normal beats
B	I	N	G	O	sudden drop in the supply of blood to an area of the heart muscle, usually due to a blockage in a coronary artery
B	I	N	G	O	inflammation of the myocardium
B	I	N	G	O	death of tissue or an organ part due to irreversible damage; usually a result of oxygen deprivation
B	I	N	G	O	the closing of a blood vessel
B	I	N	G	O	uncomfortable pulsations of the heart felt as a thumping in the chest
B	I	N	G	O	a condition at birth in which the ductus arteriousus, a small duct between the aorta and the pulmonary artery, remains abnormally open
B	I	N	G	O	lack of flow through a blood vessel, usually caused by an occlusion
B	I	N	G	O	inflammation of the pericardium
B	I	N	G	O	vascular disease in the lower extremities, usually due to the blockages in the arteries of the groin or legs
B	I	N	G	O	minute hemorrhages in the skin
B	I	N	G	O	inflammation of a vein
B	I	N	G	O	buildup of solid material, such as a fatty deposit, on the lining of an artery
B	I	N	G	O	atrial contractions that occur before the normal impulse; can be the cause of palpitations
B	I	N	G	O	ventricular contractions that occur before the normal impulse; can be the cause of palpitations
B	I	N	G	O	narrowing of the pulmonary artery, preventing the lungs from receiving enough blood from the heart to oxygenate
B	I	N	G	O	abnormal accumulation of fluid in the lungs
B	I	N	G	O	spasm in the arteries of the fingers causing numbness or pain
B	I	N	G	O	heart valve and/or muscle damage caused by an untreated streptococcal infection
B	I	N	G	O	any of various factors considered to increase the probability that a disease will occur; for example, high blood pressure and smoking are considered risk factors for heart disease
B	I	N	G	O	frictional sound heard between heartbeats, usually indication a pericardial murmur
B	I	N	G	O	hypertension having a known cause, such as kidney disease
B	I	N	G	O	congenital abnormality consisting of an opening in the septum between the atria or ventricles
B	I	N	G	O	narrowing, particularly of blood vessels or of the cardiac valves
B	I	N	G	O	heart rate greater than 100 beats per minute

B	I	N	G	O	
B	I	N	G	O	set of four congenital heart abnormalities appearing together that cause deoxygenated blood to enter the systemic circulation: ventricular septal defect, pulmonary stenosis, incorrect position of the aorta, and rich ventricular hypertrophy
B	I	N	G	O	inflammation of a vein with a thrombus
B	I	N	G	O	presence of a thrombus in a blood vessel
B	I	N	G	O	narrowing caused by a thrombus
B	I	N	G	O	stationary blood clot in the cardiovascular system, usually formed from matter found in the blood
B	I	N	G	O	abnormal narrowing of the opening of the tricuspid valve
B	I	N	G	O	inflammation of a heart valve
B	I	N	G	O	dilated, enlarged, or twisted vein, usually on the leg
B	I	N	G	O	clot on a heart valve or opening, usually caused by infection
B	I	N	G	O	surgical connection of two blood vessels to allow blood flow between them
B	I	N	G	O	opening of a blocked blood vessel, as by balloon dilation
B	I	N	G	O	viewing of the interior o f a blood vessel using a fiberoptic catheter inserted or threaded into the vessel
B	I	N	G	O	surgical incision into an artery, especially to remove a clot
B	I	N	G	O	surgical removal of an atheroma
B	I	N	G	O	insertion of a balloon catheter into a blood vessel to open the passage so blood can flow freely
B	I	N	G	O	procedure that uses a balloon catheter to open narrowed orifices in cardiac valves
B	I	N	G	O	a structure (usually a vein graft) that creates a new passage for blood flow from one artery to another artery or part of an artery; used to create a detour around blockages in the arteries
B	I	N	G	O	procedure used during surgery to divert blood flow to and from the heart through a heart- lung machine and back into circulation
B	I	N	G	O	*see angioplasty
B	I	N	G	O	*see bypass
B	I	N	G	O	surgical removal of an embolus
B	I	N	G	O	surgical removal of the diseased portion of the lining of an artery
B	I	N	G	O	any of various procedures performed during cardiac catheterization, such as angioscopy and atherectomy
B	I	N	G	O	surgical procedure that creates a bypass from the right atrium to the main pulmonary artery; fontal's procedure
B	I	N	G	O	any tissue or organ implanted to replace or mend damaged areas
B	I	N	G	O	implantation of the heart of a person who has just died into a person whose diseased heart cannot sustain life
B	I	N	G	O	surgical removal of hemorrhoids
B	I	N	G	O	stent placed within a blood vessel to allow blood to flow freely
B	I	N	G	O	*see balloon catheter dilation
B	I	N	G	O	drawing blood from a vein via a small incision
B	I	N	G	O	surgically implanted devices used to hold something (as a blood vessel) open
B	I	N	G	O	surgical removal of a thrombus
B	I	N	G	O	surgical replacement of a coronary valve
B	I	N	G	O	incision into a cardiac valve to remove an obstruction
B	I	N	G	O	surgical reconstruction of a cardiac valve
B	I	N	G	O	small puncture into a vein, usually to draw blood or inject a solution

Made in the USA
Las Vegas, NV
29 September 2024

95985196R00079